THE
PRINCETON
PLAN

THE PRINCETON PLAN

EDWIN HELENIAK, M.D.

BARBARA ASTON, M.S.

ST. MARTIN'S PRESS NEW YORK

Library of Congress Cataloging-in-Publication Data

Heleniak, Edwin.
    The Princeton plan : put your body's "good fat" to work burning away unwanted fat forever / Edwin Heleniak and Barbara Aston.
        p. cm.
    ISBN 0-312-03912-3
    1. Reducing diets.   2. Reducing exercises.   I. Aston, Barbara.
II. Title.
RM222.2 H36   1990
613.2′5—dc20   89-24140
                                                                      CIP

First Edition

10 9 8 7 6 5 4 3 2 1

NOTE TO THE READER

The menus and recipes in this book have been analyzed with the help of computer program Nutritionist III, created by N-Squared Computing Software, Salem, Oregon.

Of course, no diet can be ideal for every individual, and anyone who has a suspected medical condition, or who is taking any medication that might be affected by diet or exercise, should consult a physician before undertaking this or any other diet or exercise program.

The diet and program are the result of the authors' research and experience. Neither the publisher nor the authors makes any warranty, express or implied, with respect to this book or its contents, and neither is or shall be liable for any claims arising from use of or reliance upon this book.

For our parents
Viola and Joseph Heleniak
Elizabeth and Albert Aston,
for all their love, support, wisdom, and encouragement.
Also for
Carl C. Pfeiffer, Ph.D., M.D.,
our second father, who taught us all about nutrition.

CONTENTS

ACKNOWLEDGMENTS

We would like to express our warmest thanks to the many individuals without whose assistance this book could never have been written. We are especially grateful to Joan Carris; Jim Delo; Lynn Fellows; Larry Lynch; Christo Polycandriotis; Scott Snell; Vicki Saccardi; Doris Frechen; Petra, Heidi, and David Heleniak; Scott LaMola; the Bad-Orb Health Spa; Elizabeth Jenney; Hans Raible; Roman Lietha; Eric Braverman; Randy Gunsel; Read Hayward; Arthur Sohler; Rhoda Papaioannou; Vida Chu; Marie Arcaro; Diana Chittenden; Phyllis Loften; Sonya Friedman; Helen Hanzl; Albert Aston, Jr.; Kathryn Lance; George Grabner; and Bonnie Camo.

FOREWORD

THE preoccupation Americans have with dieting is well-known to all of us, exemplified not only by fashion magazines and television commercials, but also by the popularity of weight-loss books. At any given time, one is likely to find at least one book of this genre on the best-seller lists.

Why, then, do we need another? Because this one is different. Just as the whole concept of disease prevention through life-style modification has evolved and become mature, so has perhaps its most important component: weight control. In the past, the emphasis was on losing pounds and on achieving the appearance of being slim. This preoccupation led to a multitude of quick-weight-loss diets based on unsound principles. How many grapefruits can one eat in a day?

But despite the perception of Billy Crystal's Fernando, who reminds us that "it's better to look good than to feel good," we are now demanding both. Accordingly, weight control has become much more sophisticated, and the emphasis is where it belongs—on body composition. Almost all research linking obesity with increased risk for cardiovascular disease, cancer, and diabetes mellitus is more precisely the association between too much *fat* and these conditions, rather than too much *weight*.

In *The Princeton Plan,* Dr. Edwin Heleniak and Barbara Aston properly direct our attention to this important topic. Their creative approach to increasing metabolism by enhancing naturally and safely the body's own thermogenesis is well-grounded in scientific theory and holds great promise for many heretofore unsuccessful dieters. Their easy-to-follow diet and exercise program is geared to increasing calorie-burning lean muscle tissue and reducing calorie-storing fat, a concept that is very close to my own interests and experience.

Although no diet and exercise plan can guarantee success, if you are serious about controlling your weight, firming your muscles, and improving your health, all at the same time, *The Princeton Plan* may provide the guide you need.

—JEFFREY A. FISHER, M.D., author of
The Chromium Program

INTRODUCTION

As consumers and eaters, we are constantly bombarded with conflicting messages. We are told on the one hand that we should cut down on salt, fat, and sugar, and on the other that Americans are the best-nourished people on earth. And yet, if our diet is so good, why are such nutrition-related diseases as hypertension, diabetes, and heart disease still prevalent, accounting for billions of lost dollars a year? Why are eating disorders, such as bulimia and anorexia, practically epidemic in high schools and colleges across the country? And why are an estimated 25 percent of all Americans at least 20 percent overweight?

The sad truth is that while the diet industry makes approximately $85 billion a year, and skinny fashion models on TV and magazine covers taunt us with an impossible ideal, the prevailing culture and the standard American diet are both designed—as if deliberately—to make us fat and keep us fat!

It is not our intention in this book to attack the American food industry. But part of our purpose is to show you how and why the foods you eat—even when you are dieting—may be interfering with the proper working of your body's cells, not only preventing you from losing weight, but also encouraging you to store fat! We want to show you how your diet can influence the development of high blood pressure, diabetes, and heart disease.

Most of all we want to show you how, by making some simple changes in diet and life-style, while adding certain supplements and condiments, you can not only improve your overall health but also lose any unwanted weight and keep it off for a lifetime.

The Princeton Plan is not just another diet book, although we offer a medically proven, reduced-calorie eating plan. Rather, think of it as a guidebook through the minefield of conflicting nutritional advice, a guidebook that will show you how and what to eat not only for lasting slimness but for improved health, stamina, and lifelong well-being.

PART I

A DIETARY REVOLUTION

WHAT IS THE PRINCETON PLAN?

NOBODY ever said life is fair. But for the forty-five million Americans who are seriously overweight, the odds seem to be overwhelmingly stacked on the wrong side. After all, if there were any justice, cutting down on food would automatically result in a slow, steady loss of weight. If the world were truly fair, there wouldn't be thousands of people who can eat anything they want and never gain an ounce. If the world were fair, it wouldn't be harder to lose weight each time we try.

Traditional calorie-cutting diet books can't do anything about making the world more fair, yet they offer promises of weight loss to anyone who is willing to try them. And many of these plans do work . . . for a time. But if you are like the majority of Americans who have gone on a diet at least once in your life, you know that those lost pounds invariably creep back. Even those diets that advocate exercise as well as calorie restriction don't work for most people for the long term.

If you are a frequent dieter, then you probably read all the latest information on weight-loss research. You may already know that scientists have discovered that excess weight can be hereditary and that heavy people tend to burn calories at a slower rate than their leaner cousins. "It's all in my genes," you may be tempted to sigh. "I might as well give up." Such an attitude would be understandable—if that were the whole story. The fact is that permanent weight loss *is* attainable, for everyone, and we have written this book to show you why.

First, although there is probably a genetic component in some cases of excess weight, since it does tend to run in families, the latest cutting-edge research indicates that the lowered rate of burning calories and certain other abnormalities in overweight people are in many cases a *consequence, not a cause* of excess weight. Second, although modern diets based on setpoint theory—stressing both diet and exercise—may seem to be the last, best hope for chronic dieters, our studies clearly indicate that even these diets don't go far enough, because they address only *some* of the reasons for weight gain. In fact, until now, no diet program has been able to focus on *all* of the causes of excess weight, because not all of those causes were known.

It is only in the last few years that researchers have begun to understand fully the complexity of human weight control. And although more remains to be learned, dramatic new evidence now indicates that for many overweight people, the excess pounds are not so much a result of overeating as of an actual *defect in the body's energy production and expenditure* caused, in part, by a lifetime of eating the wrong foods. This defect not only promotes weight gain, it makes long-term weight loss virtually impossible. However, just as this and other metabolic defects were caused by bad eating habits, so they can be corrected through proper nutrition and exercise, allowing the body to burn rather than store excess calories. **The Princeton Plan is the first and only regimen that attacks fat storage on every level, actually correcting a defect in the body's ability to burn calories.**

The inability to lose excess weight is a complex problem, with external (dietary and environmental) and internal (genetic, glandular, and metabolic) causes. Only a diet that addresses *all* of these factors can work for the long term. Unlike other dietary regimens that encourage the body's tendency to slow down and conserve calories when dieting, the Princeton Plan works *with* the body, attacking excess weight on several levels. It includes:

- a balanced diet that alternates low- and high-calorie days to "fool" the body and prevent its metabolism from slowing down in response to deprivation;

- an easy-to-follow regimen that alternates low-carbohydrate days with high-carbohydrate days for maximum metabolic stimulation;

- calorie control that works by manipulating the *types* of food eaten;

- supplements and condiments that help to restore the body's natural ability to burn excess calories;

- a three-part exercise program that takes advantage of the body's own ability to "waste" calories rather than store them as fat.

THE PRINCETON PLAN AND YOU

The Princeton Plan is not hard to follow; in fact, it can seem in many ways *easier* than traditional diets because it provides the nutrition, exercise, and eating patterns your body evolved to live on. As Liz O., a Seattle-based freelance writer puts it, "The Princeton Plan is remarkably easy! It seems that I eat more than usual, but surely that isn't true." For years Liz had tried to get her boyfriend to diet. Now, with the Princeton Plan, "Ralph doesn't feel as if he's dieting. Neither one of us experiences any kind of craving, nor do we have any other complaints."

Another successful Princeton dieter, Fran C., a chiropractor and businesswoman, especially likes the alternating high- and low-carbohydrate days, because "it never gets boring like ordinary diets. Each day provides special treats," she adds. "I look forward to meat on the high-protein [i.e., low-carbohydrate] day, and bread, pasta, and beans on the high-carbo day."

Unlike fad diets, there are sound scientific reasons behind every element of the Princeton Plan, reasons appreciated by veteran dieters. "This is the first diet plan that made scientific sense to me," says Shirley M., a sixty-one-year-old medical administrative assistant. "Maybe that's why it's the first one that's worked."

Nancy K., an epidemiologist, agrees. "A diet is much more than just food," she says. "The Princeton Plan translates scientific information into hope."

You needn't be a medical professional to understand the theories behind the Princeton Plan. In the pages that follow, we will explain exactly how it works on the whole body as well as at the cellular level. We will show you why it must work for you and will help you to lose weight and keep it off. For perhaps the first time in your life, you will receive the complete nutrition your body needs to function properly. The Princeton Plan can help you feel better than you ever have.

In Parts II, III, and IV you will find step-by-step directions for following the Princeton Plan, including sample menus, recipes, and tips on making the Plan a part of your life. We will show you in detail how to incorporate our three-part exercise program, which takes just minutes a day, into your routine to streamline your body.

Appendixes A through D contain instructions for customizing the diet to your own metabolism and food preferences; a selected bibliography gives suggestions for further reading.

Appendix E consists of an abstract from our original scientific paper outlining our plan, and is intended for professional workers in the fields of nutrition and obesity.

If you're anxious to get started on the Princeton Plan, by all means skip to Part II and begin. But we hope you will come back and read Part I so you will understand all the reasons for our recommendations—and so you will never again be tempted to follow an unhealthful crash diet that cheats your body of the nutrients it needs and guarantees continued poundage and an unhealthy life.

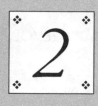

THE METABOLIC TRAP

A NOTE ON CALORIES AND ENERGY

EVEN if you've never been on a diet, you have certainly heard about calories. If you're a veteran of the weight-loss wars, you have probably counted them and memorized the calorie content of your favorite foods—but you still may not know exactly what calories are. Simply put, a calorie is a unit of energy; specifically, the amount of heat energy that it takes to raise 1 gram of water (less than a thimbleful) by 1 degree Celsius. (In nutritional terms, a Calorie, also called a *kilocalorie*, is equal to 1,000 calories.)

Energy, in chemical and physical terms, can exist in several forms: It can be stored (all fuels are stored forms of energy); and it can be expended in motion, in chemical and electrical processes, or as heat. When you eat, you ingest energy stored in the form of food and then use it in a number of ways: in chemical processes, such as digestion; in motion (jogging, dialing a telephone); in converting it to heat; or by storing it, as fat or glycogen (a form of starch).

In explaining how our Plan works, we will be talking about *calories* and *energy*. Throughout, bear in mind that these are really two ways of talking about the same thing.

A DIETARY REVOLUTION

If you are like most dieters, you have tried to lose weight over and over—and sometimes you have succeeded. But always, eventually, the weight has crept back, seemingly with a mind of its own. The sad fact is that, along with countless other dieters, you have a body that has become too efficient. It's too efficient at digesting foods, and it's too efficient at converting them to fat. It simply won't use up extra calories, no matter how much you might like it to. This trait would have been quite useful in caveman days, when periodic famine was a fact of life. But today, unfortunately, your metabolic efficiency leaves you with unwanted pounds and a susceptibility to the diseases associated with excess weight, such as diabetes and hypertension.

Although you have probably known for most of your life that it is hard for you to lose weight on a calorie-restricted diet, most experts in the diet field did not agree with you, until fairly recently. In fact, it's only in the last decade or so that serious attention has been paid to individual differences in the ability to lose or gain weight. And it's only the very latest research that has made possible the revolutionary ideas that combine to form the Princeton Plan.

The principles behind our Plan seem to be revolutionary because in the past, most research into the causes of excess weight has been based on faulty, though seemingly logical, assumptions. For many years, experts on obesity "knew" that weight loss was a simple matter of arithmetic. Energy taken in, in the form of calories, had to equal energy expended—through the processes of living and in physical activity. If the two sides of the equation didn't match, the result was an energy imbalance: When the amount was greater on the intake side, weight would be gained; on the output side, weight lost.

Thus, since one pound is equivalent to approximately 3,500 calories of stored energy, to lose that pound you would have to reduce food intake by 3,500 calories. Cutting out one hundred calories a day should, in theory, result in the loss of one pound in thirty-five days. Because this equation seemed so straightforward, early diets were designed to limit the intake of food; with the remaining part of the equation—the output—presumed unchanged, the logical result should be weight loss. Until fairly recently, nearly all popular diets (such as the Scarsdale Diet) were essentially calorie-restricted diets. Unfortunately, simple calorie restriction didn't work for many dieters, who failed either to lose weight on such a regimen or to keep it off.

Because calorie restriction proved so unsuccessful for so many dieters, a rash of nutritionally poor fad diets (such as the various low-carbohydrate diets and the Beverly Hills Diet) tempted those looking for a miracle. These unbalanced diets generally caused quick water loss, thus seeming to work for a time, but they were too lacking in nutrition to follow on a long-term basis, and most dieters quickly regained any lost pounds. While most responsible doctors recommended getting more exercise, few seriously considered this to be a good way to lose weight, because of what *seemed* to be a discouraging mathematical reality: The numbers indicated that only huge amounts of exercise could make a difference—walking 35 miles, for example, to burn off 1 pound of fat.

It was not until the late 1970s that researchers began to reexamine the energy balance and to realize that while the equation is fundamentally correct, it fails to take into account individual differences among dieters and the metabolic effects of exercise. While in theory almost anyone should lose weight on 1,000 calories per day, many people don't. In the past, the doctors who counseled such unfortunate dieters assumed their clients were cheating on their diets. When researchers began to focus on the output side of the energy equation, however, they discovered some surprising facts. For one thing, studies began to appear showing that most overweight people are less active than their lean cousins. It was also found that diet and exercise combined in a synergistic effect that counted for more than just the energy cost of the activity, and that this combination was thus far more effective in weight loss than diet alone. These studies concluded, therefore, that a successful diet should focus not only on reducing the input (calorie restriction) but at the same time on increasing the output (energy expenditure). This new emphasis on activity was a step in the right direction. Such books as *The Dieter's Dilemma* and *The Setpoint Diet,* advocating exercise as well as calorie restriction, began to hit the best-seller lists.

But for large numbers of dieters, the new approach was still not as effective as it might have been. Too many dieters still could not lose as much weight as they wanted to, or would lose it and quickly regain it. The new diet-and-exercise regimens were far more successful than the old calorie-restricted approach, but even these new diets still focused on only a small part of the energy equation. Although they increased the dieter's energy expenditure through activity, the plans did not affect the biggest component of the body's energy output. The truth is that for most people, exercise (including daily activity as well as sports and calisthenics) accounts for only 12 percent of total energy expenditure.

The remaining 88 percent of energy expended by your body is produced by **resting metabolism** (the energy used in all living processes, such as breathing, digestion, tissue repair, and so on) and by **thermogenesis**, literally, heat production. Animal and human studies have all shown that the very act of cutting food intake causes the body to decrease *both* these sources of energy expenditure. Thus, dieters are caught in a neat trap: The more they cut down on food intake, the more their bodies reduce energy production. And even when they succeed in losing weight, studies show that formerly fat people continue to burn calories 15 percent slower than normal-weight people. No wonder so many people have found lasting weight loss unattainable!

It is only very recently that science has begun to show a way out of this metabolic trap. By combining theories from a number of different researchers in several fields, we have created a multifaceted program that at last directly affects that 88 percent of your body's energy production. Our program increases both resting metabolic rate and thermogenesis, not only preventing the downturn in metabolism that accompanies ordinary diets but actually increasing the number of calories you burn all day long.

WHY TRADITIONAL DIETS FAIL

We will explain in detail all facets of the Princeton Plan in later chapters, but first we want to give a brief explanation of why traditional diets seldom work for the long term. Most of these diets take into account only one side of the energy equation; and many of them perpetuate the unhealthy cravings and food addictions that helped make you overweight in the first place. Furthermore, virtually all popular diets are deficient in certain essential nutrients, and no diet can work in the long run unless it can be the basis for a lifelong eating plan.

Some well-known diets can even compromise your health. For

example, low-carbohydrate, high-protein diets, such as Scarsdale, can cause kidney damage, and their lack of fiber promotes constipation and can increase cholesterol. The even more restrictive liquid-protein diets have led to electrolyte imbalance and even death. None of these diets can form the basis for a long-time dietary plan, because of the health consequences and the monotony.

The low-carbohydrate, high-fat diets, such as the Stillman Diet and the Drinking Man's Diet, are also dangerous; their lack of balanced nutrition and high saturated-fat content can worsen the condition of anyone with diabetes or heart disease.

Safer are the high-carbohydrate, low-fat regimens, including Pritikin and macrobiotic diets, but even with very careful food selection it is difficult to obtain all needed nutrients on these plans. Also, because these diets have very low fat content, few people accustomed to a Western diet can stick to them for more than a few days. The biggest problem with these diets is that they make it difficult to obtain enough of the fats that, as we will explain later, are essential for the proper working of all body systems.

Finally, there are numerous fad diets, such as the Beverly Hills Diet and the Grapefruit Diet, which usually rely on a gimmick, such as the myth that some food or combination of foods can "burn off" fat. Not only is this completely false—no food can burn off fat directly—it can also be very dangerous to follow such diets for any length of time, because they are so lacking in essential nutrients.

Which brings us to one of the greatest difficulties with all traditional diets: Any diet that restricts calories is also bound to be deficient in micronutrients, the substances that your body needs in very small amounts for proper functioning. In fact, it is partly the absence of these nutrients that dooms most diets to failure. When your body does not receive the nutrition it needs, it signals you with hunger pangs, which can lead to irritability, feelings of deprivation, and, ultimately, bingeing or otherwise going off the diet. Furthermore—and even worse news for anyone who is trying to lose weight—some of these micronutrients are essential for the proper functioning of the body's fat storage and burning system. If these are missing in the diet, then the metabolism is further slowed, and excess fat cannot be burned.

The Princeton Plan, based on the very latest medical and nutritional research, provides complete nutrition. It avoids the drawbacks that have doomed earlier diets to failure, while at the same time ensuring that all systems of your body function properly for the fastest and steadiest weight loss possible. Rather than concentrating on total calories, or grams of carbohydrate, or portions, we focus on the nutrients themselves.

Most important, the Princeton Plan addresses every facet of weight loss, from the metabolic to the behavioral. To see how it works, let's take a look at what goes on in your body when you ingest food.

THE MISSING LINKS

IN the days when dieting was considered essentially a matter of mathematical balance, no one thought seriously about the connection between the type of energy intake and the type of output. It was assumed to be a more or less automatic, mathematical process. If you ate an extra 100 calories, whether those calories came from chocolate or lettuce, your body would store them as fat, unless you did 100 calories worth of exercise (say, walked a mile) to burn them off. New studies on energy balance have shown, however, that this notion is false. The type of food you eat can spell the difference between weight gain and weight loss, as can the type of exercise you get and when you exercise in relation to your meals.

The truth is that the system controlling **energy balance** in the body is far more complex than early scientists imagined. As with other body systems, each part is closely linked to every other part, and all links are essential for the proper functioning of the whole. A weak or missing link can cause the entire system to proceed inefficiently or fail, resulting in energy imbalance and weight gain. In this chapter we will take a look at each of the links in this "chain" and the ways in which they can malfunction; in the next chapter we will examine some of the behavioral and nutritional strategies that can help to restore proper energy balance.

SETPOINT AND METABOLISM

In the early 1980s nutritionists and doctors who worked with chronic dieters began to develop a concept known as **setpoint theory**. Briefly, this theory states that just as your body uses a number of strategies (for example, shivering and sweating) to maintain a constant temperature, it also uses a number of strategies to maintain a constant weight. Each of us, this theory holds, has a "preferred" weight that the body will vigorously try to defend. Thus, if your natural setpoint is 140 pounds, you will find it difficult to diet down to 125 pounds. You will also find it hard to gain, permanently, even a few ounces. Even worse, once you manage to lose, say, 15 pounds, your body will do everything it can to see that you quickly regain that lost weight.

Although there is some doubt about whether a literal setpoint exists, it is certain that our bodies resist sudden significant weight change and that naturally skinny people find it just as difficult to gain weight as fat people do to lose it. It is also well known that there are marked individual differences in the ability to gain or lose weight. While some people can eat three cheeseburgers at a time with impunity, others seem to gain weight just by "looking" at a slice of cake. Although not everything is yet known about the reasons for these individual differences, researchers have demonstrated that they are initiated in the very cells of our bodies, where energy is created and stored.

To get a better understanding of these complex processes and how they affect your weight, let's start with the three ways in which your body can expend energy, or burn calories. These are physical activity, resting metabolism, and thermogenesis. Although resting metabolism and thermogenesis are not completely separate processes, it is convenient to consider them separately. **Physical activity**, which includes all voluntary activity from calisthenics to fidgeting, usually accounts for 12 percent of all the energy you expend. Metabolism and thermogenesis together account for the other 88 percent.

Resting metabolism is the term for the energy you use when resting quietly, several hours after a meal or exercise. It includes all the processes that keep your body alive: the energy expended in pumping blood, maintaining body temperature, exchanging oxygen and carbon dioxide, digesting and storing food, repairing and creating new cells, and fighting infections. All of these are part of your resting metabolism, and all are known as **metabolic processes.**

Thermogenesis, on the other hand, is the mechanism that allows your metabolism to eliminate rather than store or use calories. Literally, it means "heat production," and the body calls on it whenever it is necessary to dispose of unwanted calories or generate extra heat in cold temperatures.

THERMOGENESIS AND BAT

Because thermogenesis can eliminate excess energy, researchers have long suspected it plays a role in successful weight loss and, indeed, the latest studies indicate that it is the *key* to lasting weight loss. The key to thermogenesis, in turn, is a specialized body tissue known as brown fat—or, as it is called in the scientific literature, **BAT (brown adipose tissue).** BAT is located primarily at the back of the neck and between the shoulder blades, as well as around vital organs, including the heart and kidneys.

BAT has been studied extensively in rats and other small mammals. Like ordinary white fat cells, BAT cells store fat molecules. But unlike white fat, BAT does not make us "fat." Its main function in the body, through a complex series of biochemical reactions, is to convert its fat stores to heat. It is BAT's ability to produce heat that keeps newborn baby mammals, including humans, warm when they emerge from the womb. The activation of BAT is what allows some animals to hibernate through the winter without freezing; the same mechanism also allows animals to overeat when food is plentiful without becoming fat. The excess calories from such feasts are literally burned up.

Numerous experiments have now confirmed that in several strains of genetically obese rats, the reason for the obesity is a defect in thermogenesis: The rat is lacking the proper amount of BAT or its body is unable to activate BAT. Rats with normally functioning BAT are seldom obese. In one experiment, for instance, rats kept in a cold environment were able to eat two times the normal amount of food without gaining an ounce; clearly, their BAT was using the extra calories to keep them warm.

Emerging studies are beginning to focus on thermogenesis in humans, and it is becoming ever-clearer that defective thermogenesis—due either to insufficient or improperly functioning BAT—is largely responsible for excess poundage and the inability to lose weight.

In fact, excess weight itself sabotages the ability of BAT to function, which leads to further weight gain, in a truly vicious circle. And dieting suppresses BAT even more. It seems obvious, then, that **the key to permanent weight loss is to increase the amount or the activity of BAT**, but until recently too little was known about thermogenesis in humans to make this possible.

It is only in the last few years that researchers have unlocked the complex biochemical pathways by which BAT works to create thermogenesis. In fact, because humans contain much less BAT proportionately than rats, it was not known for certain until fairly recently that adult humans even possessed BAT. New research has demonstrated, however, that they do indeed possess BAT and that it plays an important role in thermogenesis. In fact, a very small amount of human BAT—less than one-tenth of 1 percent of body weight—can make a difference of up to 20 to 25 percent in metabolic rate. **It is undoubtedly the presence and activity of BAT that accounts for wide individual differences in the ability to gain or lose weight.**

It is now believed that many, if not all, overweight people may not possess sufficient BAT or may be unable to activate it properly. Although thermogenesis itself is fairly straightforward—"burning" fatty molecules to produce heat—it can happen only after a specific series of physiological events occurs, and the process can break down anywhere along the line.

HOW BAT WORKS TO CREATE
THERMOGENESIS

Although the end product—heat—is the same, thermogenesis occurs in either of two circumstances: in response to food or in response to cold.

The first kind of thermogenesis is called **dietary-induced thermogenesis**, and it consists of two components. The first, which occurs every time we eat, is the heat produced as a by-product of the digestion, transport, and storage of food. Physiologists refer to this form of thermogenesis as **obligatory** thermogenesis, and it accounts for as much as 10 percent of the caloric value of a food.

The second component of dietary-induced thermogenesis consists of the heat produced when excess calories—those in excess of what the body needs to maintain itself—are burned, or "wasted." This form of thermogenesis is referred to as **adaptive**, and it takes place entirely within BAT tissue. The optimum production of adaptive thermogenesis depends on the types of food eaten and other factors, starting with the sympathetic nervous system.

THE SYMPATHETIC NERVOUS SYSTEM

Although it sounds as if it must have something to do with the emotions, your sympathetic nervous system consists of nerves that control the functioning of many of your inner organs, including your heart, lungs, and intestinal tract. It is responsible for maintaining body temperature and other critical life functions, as well as revving up body systems to meet emergencies. The sympathetic nervous system also helps to regulate appetite and the storage of fat. When the sympathetic nervous system is stimulated, it secretes norepinephrine, a neurotransmitter that raises the metabolism. Neurotransmitters are the chemical "languages" used by the brain for communication within the brain and between the brain and the rest of the nervous system. There are about fifty such languages. The amino acids, building blocks of proteins, make up most neurotransmitters. When the sympathetic nerves within BAT tissue secrete norepinephrine, a biochemical reaction results in oxidation, or "burning" of fat molecules. Since it is responsible for activating BAT, the sympathetic nervous system is critical in maintaining both normal body weight and temperature. In fact, certain strains of obese rats that are unable to respond to norepinephrine freeze to death when put into a cold environment.

It is now known that **food restriction itself diminishes sympathetic-nervous-system activity, lowering the metabolic rate.** Thus, the very act of dieting reduces the amount of norepinephrine available to your body, forcing it to conserve the few calories that you take in. This slowing of the body's natural fires begins within twenty-four to forty-eight hours of caloric restriction and actually increases the longer the diet continues.

Clearly, any successful diet must encourage activity of the sympathetic nervous system, for proper stimulation of metabolism and of BAT. And this is where the composition of a diet becomes crucial: In order for the sympathetic nervous system to function optimally, your body must have certain nutrients available. Among the most important of these are essential fatty acids.

ESSENTIAL FATTY ACIDS

Among the most important links in the chain leading to thermogenesis are **essential fatty acids (EFAs),** long molecules that are the building blocks of certain fats. Fatty acids are found in every cell of the body and are responsible, among other things, for providing energy, insulating nerves, and cushioning and protecting cells and organs. *Essential* fatty acids are so called because they must be supplied by diet; the body cannot make them. Current research has established that essential fatty acids play a central role in regulating appetite and maintaining weight. Studies show, for example, that **when the body does not get enough of the essential fatty acids, appetite increases,** perhaps in an attempt to try to supply the missing nutrients. Conversely, lab animals on a diet high in essential fatty acids are less likely than animals on a standard diet to become fat.

In a study in which humans were given a large excess of calories in combination with a supplement containing essential fatty acids, most of the volunteers lost weight despite the extra calories. They also reported feeling hot and sweating, indicating that the excess calories were being burned off.

It wasn't until fairly recently that we learned *how* essential fatty acids help stimulate thermogenesis, and numerous studies now show that their action is indirect; along with other nutrients they are precursors—necessary building blocks—of prostaglandins, the next link in the chain leading to thermogenesis. (For more information on essential fatty acids and other fatty acids, see chapter 5.)

PROSTAGLANDINS

You may have read about **prostaglandins**, which are similar to hormones and which are currently a hot topic in medical circles. Unlike hormones, which are produced in one part of the body but act on another part (like insulin), prostaglandins are manufactured by each organ for its own immediate use. Various prostaglandins are responsible for nearly every activity in your body, including dilation and constriction of blood vessels, regulation of temperature, muscle contraction (including contractions of the uterus), fighting off infections, and many other processes. Prostaglandins tend to come in pairs. For example, if one prostaglandin causes inflammation, another reduces it. After performing its assigned function, a prostaglandin is immediately destroyed; these powerful chemicals are constantly being made and unmade. **A number of prostaglandins are active not only in thermogenesis but also in the control of appetite and regulation of fat tissue. Without sufficient essential fatty acids in the diet, the necessary prostaglandins cannot be made, and thermogenesis cannot take place.**

INSULIN

Another key link in the chain leading to thermogenesis is **insulin**. You probably know that this hormone, manufactured in the pancreas, is responsible for maintaining a constant level of sugar in your blood. In a healthy body, insulin attaches itself to special receptors on muscle cells and in the liver, allowing the cells to "open up" after a meal and take in excess sugar from the bloodstream. But if there isn't enough insulin, or if it can't attach to the receptors, the level of sugar in the blood rises and serious health consequences, including diabetes, can result.

Insulin is involved in other body processes as well. Numerous studies have demonstrated that it must be present for dietary-induced thermogenesis to occur, that it stimulates the sympathetic nervous system, and that it is responsible for helping to "turn on" BAT after overeating. Unfortunately, many, if not all, overweight people have a condition called **insulin resistance**, in which their insulin does not function properly because it either cannot attach itself to insulin receptors or because there are not enough receptors. The result is impaired thermogenesis, and an actual increase in body fat, because high levels of insulin in the blood promote fat storage. Furthermore, insulin resistance leads to water retention, which causes bloating and can contribute to high blood pressure.

Although researchers believed for years that insulin resistance was a *cause* of excess weight, the opposite is now believed to be true: i.e., that excess weight in itself actually causes insulin resistance. It's not known exactly how, but researchers speculate that it may come about from frequent snacking on high-sugar or high-fat foods, which prevents insulin from returning to normal levels. Also, there is evidence that a diet high in animal fats promotes insulin resistance.

Insulin resistance is not uncommon, but luckily there are a number of ways to overcome it, including proper diet, exercise, and weight loss itself.

OTHER FACTORS

In addition to the factors mentioned above, there are many others that affect energy balance in the body. Nearly all of them work by increasing the amount of BAT or its activation through the sympathetic nervous system. Particularly important are a number of hormones, including thyroid, human growth hormone, and melatonin, which is produced by the pineal gland in response to shortened periods of light and increased cold. We will discuss the role of these and other factors later in the book.

THERMOGENESIS IN RESPONSE TO COLD

The second type of thermogenesis is called **nonshivering thermogenesis** (it is so named because shivering involves physical movement, generating heat in muscle tissue). In fact, **the mere presence of a cold environment seems to stimulate growth of BAT, and when coupled with exercise, it stimulates it even more.** Studies have shown greater-than-average BAT deposits in Finnish outdoor workers and Korean pearl divers, who ply their trade in icy waters.

THE EXERCISE CONNECTION

It has been well known for several years that any diet is more effective when combined with exercise. Recent research has explained why that is true and points to strategies that take advantage of all the ways in which exercise can help initiate and maintain weight loss.

1. Exercise burns calories. This seems obvious, but while exercise accounts for only 12 percent of energy expenditure in sedentary adults, that amount can easily be increased, through programmed whole-body exercises as well as "life-style" exercises—ways of adding more activity to the day. (See Part II for detailed, easy-to-follow instructions for a three-part exercise program.)

2. Exercise raises metabolism and increases dietary-induced thermogenesis for up to twelve to eighteen hours. Studies have shown that the resting metabolism is similar in lean and heavy people. But dietary-induced thermogenesis is significantly lower in the overweight. Since dietary-induced thermogenesis accounts for 5 to 10 percent of total energy expenditure, it is no wonder that so many people have difficulty losing weight! The good news is that **exercise *before* meals can actually increase dietary-induced thermogenesis in overweight people. Furthermore, regular exercise can increase the resting metabolism for extended periods of time.** In one study, overweight women were divided into two groups; one group just dieted, while the other combined exercise and dieting. At the end of three months, those in the group that had exercised were thinner and had a 12 percent higher resting metabolism.

    This is encouraging news for anyone trying to lose weight. It appears that exercise itself uses calories, and it actually helps you to burn more calories *all day long,* no matter what you are doing. In fact, it has been estimated that the true energy "cost" of exercise is up to two times higher than the energy used for the actual activity.

3. Traditional diets that do not include exercise destroy muscle, while exercise builds muscle. Studies show that the weight lost with calorie restriction alone consists of 75 percent fat and 25 percent muscle; when exercise is added, only 5 percent of the

weight lost is muscle tissue. This effect speeds further weight loss, since muscle tissue is more metabolically active than fat tissue, meaning that it takes more calories to maintain it. The greater the percentage of muscle in your body, the more calories you will burn all the time. Furthermore, muscle tissue is heavier than fat tissue, but it takes up less space, so a more muscular body looks slimmer than a fat one, even if no weight is lost.

4.   Intangible benefits. Although this cannot be quantified scientifically, the very act of doing regular exercise makes you feel better, physically and psychologically. You will have increased energy because your body systems will become more efficient. And as an added bonus, for most people regular exercise decreases appetite.

PUTTING IT ALL TOGETHER

The Princeton Plan is the first and only diet that works with your body, using its own processes to ensure successful weight loss. On the Plan, you will learn how to manipulate your diet, life-style, and activity level to:

- maximize thermogenesis by stimulating and increasing BAT;

- maximize your metabolic rate;

- increase your muscle mass.

In the next two chapters we will explain in more detail how the Princeton Plan works, and in Part II we will provide step-by-step instructions.

HOW THE PRINCETON
PLAN WORKS

ALTHOUGH humans may not seem to have much in common with rodents, rats are used widely in laboratory nutrition studies because many of their digestive and metabolic processes are similar to ours. Yet, except for certain strains of rats that are specially bred to be fat, researchers know that it is difficult to get rats to overeat and gain weight. It is difficult, that is, unless the rats are fed a special diet known as the "supermarket" or "cafeteria" diet, a diet that is very similar to the typical American diet, consisting of such varied, delicious, and high-fat items as cheese, peanut butter, chocolate, salami, and the like.

These foods are all high in calories, and their composition is such that they are readily stored as fat. Furthermore, they are lacking vital nutrients that, in a more natural diet, would help a rat—or human—stay slim.

What supermarket-fed rats (and many of us) are eating are truly "empty calories." The calories are considered empty because, while they contain *energy,* they are virtually devoid of the micronutrients we need for the proper working of our bodies on a cellular level. Left to their own devices, rats won't eat such nutrition-poor food. Studies have established, for example, that neither rats nor cockroaches will eat white flour when alternatives are available. Unfortunately, humans seem to have lost such natural nutritional wisdom: A recent survey found that the average American eats 12 pounds of potato chips annually, compared to 3 pounds of broccoli. The shocking fact is that two-thirds of the calories in a typical American diet come from highly processed foods such as refined carbohydrates, purified fats and oils, and alcohol, which cannot possibly provide the complete nutrition of the whole foods from which they were extracted.

Traditional diets, even those advocating exercise, that are based primarily on calorie restriction give little attention to the form those calories take. **In the Princeton Plan, the *type* of calories eaten is one of the most important—and most effective—parts of the regimen.** We insist on a diet of whole foods—what you may think of as "health foods." This is so for a very good reason. Any diet that is calorie-restricted will, by definition, be nutrient-restricted, too. Even very tiny amounts of certain substances, when missing from the diet, can make a big difference to the overall health of the body; and, for our purposes, they can also make a big difference in the body's ability to stimulate thermogenesis effectively.

In the Princeton Plan *every* calorie counts. Instead of "empty" calories, we provide calories that are packed with nutrients. We also recommend a variety of supplements and condiments to make certain that the diet contains every micronutrient essential for proper thermogenesis and metabolic functions as well as those necessary for overall health. None of these supplements is in any way exotic or toxic.

Foods recommended in the Princeton Plan include whole grains and products made from them (breads, pasta, cereals, etc.), fresh vegetables (raw, steamed, in soups and salads), fresh fruits, nuts and seeds, dried peas and beans, low-fat dairy products, eggs, lean meats, poultry (without skin), and fish and shellfish. Beverages include pure tap water, mineral water, bottled water, seltzer, sugar-free fruit juices, herbal teas, coffee and tea, grain coffee substitutes, and skim, 1- or 2-percent milk. Oils, spices, herbs, and lemon juice may be used for flavoring. The only foods not allowed are those that have had their nutrition "processed" out of them: refined sugar and white flour and products made from them (candy, cakes, cookies); and products high in saturated fat such as hot dogs, luncheon meats, and foods cooked in lard. Some foods forbidden on many traditional diets, such as red meat and butter, are permitted in small amounts, as is alcohol, as long as it is used sparingly.

A final note. For various reasons the terms *health food* and *whole food* have an ambiguous and even shady reputation in the popular press. Many Americans assume that such foods are bland or boring: "rabbit food," made from exotic or bad-tasting ingredients. Others fear that eating whole foods must mean tedious hours of cooking from scratch or foraging for nuts and berries. Let us set you at ease on both counts. Whole foods include many of the foods that you most enjoy now, including whole-grain breads and pastas, meat, and eggs. The main difference is that you will prepare your meals with less oil, fat, and salt than you are accustomed to and that you will use complex-carbohydrate ingredients instead of refined ones. It is true that some whole foods, such as brown rice, take longer to cook than their denatured, processed alternatives (e.g., white rice). But you should also note that there are many shortcuts even in using whole foods: Quick-cooking brown rice, for example, cooks faster than any white rice except the pasty, tasteless "instant" variety; and there are many healthful canned and frozen products including beans, vegetables, and fruits.

These and other shortcuts are emphasized in our menu and recipe section, beginning on page 103.

EATING AND EXERCISING TO MAXIMIZE WEIGHT LOSS

In Part II of this book, we will give you simple, step-by-step instructions for following the Princeton Plan. But for now we want to explain exactly why each element is included and what it does. Bear in mind that all parts of the plan are interrelated and that **the goal of each part of the Princeton Plan is to help you burn as many calories as possible while following a healthy eating and exercise plan.**

1. The Princeton Plan Stimulates Metabolism Through Manipulation of Dietary Composition

Apart from a few fad diets that emphasize one or two types of food (say, fats and proteins), or are based on only one food, such as the Grapefruit Diet, most diets emphasize cutting calories, period.

Interestingly, however, the *composition* of the diet, the relative amounts of protein, carbohydrate, and fat, as well as the types of each, have been proven to have an effect on body weight as least as important as, and perhaps more so than, the total caloric intake of food.

- **High levels of carbohydrate have been proven to stimulate the sympathetic nervous system and thus enhance thermogenesis.** In a study of vegetarians, volunteers who began to eat beef were found to have lower norepinephrine levels after only four weeks, a sign of diminished sympathetic-nervous-system activity and lower overall metabolism. The Princeton Plan emphasizes complex carbohydrates to a greater extent than most weight-loss diets and much more than the standard American diet.

- **All calories are not alike.** The energy cost of converting carbohydrate to fat and storing it is 23 percent of each calorie; the cost of storing a calorie of fat is only 3 percent of that calorie. Thus, for every carbohydrate calorie eaten, nearly 25 percent is "wasted" in metabolic processes, while a fat calorie is, as the old joke goes, "applied directly to your hips." A study by researchers at the U.S. Department of Agriculture found that women who cut their fat intake from 40 percent to 20 percent, but kept their total calorie intake the same, lost 1 percent of their body fat after four months.

   For maximum stimulation of the metabolism, then, our plan consists of 55 percent complex carbohydrate, 20 percent protein, and 25 percent fat, when averaged over the two-day alternating plan.

- **Day-to-day composition of the diet affects the metabolism.** In chapter 3, we saw that the metabolic rate begins to fall within twenty-four to forty-eight hours of calorie restriction. As dieting continues, metabolism falls even further, resulting in the well-known "plateau effect."

   Strangely, however, studies show that short-term *overeating* can also stimulate the sympathetic nervous system and initiate thermogenesis. (This explains why dietary-induced thermogenesis increases in normal-weight people after an unusually heavy meal.) In both cases sympathetic activity (metabolism) returns quickly to normal as soon as food intake returns to accustomed levels.

These metabolic effects, which may be strategies from the days when our remote ancestors literally faced feast or famine on a continual basis, can be put to work to "fool" the body and help speed weight loss.

In the Princeton Plan, we recommend a diet that alternates the number of calories taken in every other day. Day 1 of the diet acts as the calorie-cutting day, with its emphasis on low-carbohydrate complete-protein foods such as eggs, lean meat, poultry, and fish. Day 2 of the diet, with its high carbohydrate and higher calorie content, counteracts the metabolic slow-down that occurs as a result of Day 1, when calories are cut. This system provides optimal stimulation of the sympathetic nervous system and hence thermogenesis, without slowing the metabolism, as commonly happens on ordinary diets. Thus, on the Princeton Plan you can avoid the plateau effect that occurs when metabolism slows as a result of calorie restriction, *and* you can actually stimulate the metabolism to speed the burning of calories. Furthermore, because the diet alternates from day to day, it is more interesting than a diet that offers the same basic plan every day.

• **Short-term changes in the percentage of carbohydrate consumed stimulate metabolism.** The Princeton Plan diet alternates on a two-day basis as follows:

Low-calorie, low-carbohydrate day: 45% carbohydrate
25% protein
30% fat
High-calorie, high-carbohydrate day: 65% carbohydrate
15% protein
20% fat

For men on a 1500-calorie diet, this works out to 1200 calories offered one day, and 1700 calories the next. For women on a 1200-calorie diet, the regimen alternates between 1000-calorie and 1400-calorie days.

Averaged over a two-day period, this diet is very nutritious and closely matches the U.S. Senate Select Committee on Nu-

trition and Human Needs recommendation for 55 percent carbohydrate, 30 percent fat, and 15 percent protein. (We offer
slightly higher amounts of protein because weight reduction
and increased exercise both increase the need for protein.)

- **Some fats are essential for weight loss and good health.** The
Princeton Plan is a low-fat diet compared to the standard American diet. It does, however, emphasize the importance of the
essential fatty acids, which are vital for weight loss and good
health. In addition, fat adds what nutritionists call "palatabil-
ity," or flavor and texture. Very few people who are used to a
Western diet can easily give up those enhancements and stick
to a very low-fat plan for the long term.

   Second, as we saw in chapter 3, essential fatty acids are
found *only* in certain oils. Essential fatty acids are essential for
proper metabolism and appetite control, and, as precursors to
prostaglandins, they are one of the key links in the chain that
ends in thermogenesis.

   The Princeton Plan, then, emphasizes *specific* fats and oils.
Of the 20 to 30 percent fat allowed in the diet, approximately
10 percent is polyunsaturated, 5 to 10 percent monounsaturated, and 5 to 10 percent saturated. These fats and oils are
obtained through seeds, nuts, certain vegetable oils, fatty fish,
and supplements. (For more information on fats and oils, see
chapter 5.)

2. The Princeton Plan Helps Restore Insulin Sensitivity

The Princeton Plan works in several ways to help restore insulin
sensitivity, thus increasing dietary-induced thermogenesis and inhibit-
ing fat formation.

- **Weight loss itself tends to restore insulin sensitivity.**

- **Dietary composition affects insulin sensitivity.** In the
Princeton Plan, we employ a number of dietary strategies to
correct insulin resistance. These include cutting back on animal
fats, which in excess can lead to carbohydrate intolerance; eliminating refined carbohydrates, which elevate levels of insulin;
reducing the intake of salt, which increases sugar in the blood

and thus raises insulin levels; and increasing fiber, which helps
both to normalize insulin metabolism and eliminate constipation.

- **Regular exercise has been shown to restore normal insulin
  functioning.**

- **Prostaglandins are essential for normal insulin tolerance.**
  The Princeton Plan offers selected supplements to ensure that
  all prostaglandin precursors are included in the diet.

3. The Princeton Plan Stimulates BAT, Increasing Thermogenesis

Since we now know that a major reason for the failure of so many
people to lose weight on a long-term basis is defective thermogenesis,
any weight-loss program should aim at increasing and stimulating
BAT. In the Princeton Plan we do this in a number of ways:

- **Eating stimulates thermogenesis.** Dietary-induced thermogenesis—the energy "cost" of eating, digesting, and storing
  foods—lasts for several hours after a meal. In fact, eating itself
  raises the resting metabolism by 10 to 35 percent and accounts
  for 5 to 10 percent of total energy expenditure. In the Princeton Plan we take advantage of this natural stoking of the body's
  fires by emphasizing small, frequent meals throughout the day.
  Studies have shown that the same number of calories, eaten all
  in one meal, are more readily stored as fat than those eaten in
  several smaller meals. This form of "grazing" has another advantage as well, in helping to keep the dieter from feeling
  hunger and being tempted to go off the diet or binge.

- **Exercise stimulates thermogenesis.** Pound for pound, resting metabolism is similar in the lean and the overweight. But
  dietary-induced thermogenesis is lower in heavier people. It is,
  however, increased by exercise, especially when the exercise
  occurs before a meal. Exercising before eating has another
  advantage: For most people it will reduce appetite. The con-
  verse is true as well: Rats, when deprived of exercise, respond
  with a greater appetite.

- **Thermogenic nutrients stimulate BAT.** In addition to increasing resting metabolic rate, a diet high in complex carbohy-

drates also stimulates the sympathetic nervous system and therefore BAT activity. A number of supplements can also have a
thermogenic effect; see page 31.

- **Cold exposure stimulates thermogenesis.** BAT is stimulated
  by two things: food and cold, especially cold coupled with
  exercise. Our plan recommends exercising in the cold, using
  cold towels or packs, and taking cold showers. For full details,
  see chapter 19.

*4. The Princeton Plan Increases Energy Expenditure Through Timing of and
Alternating Types of Exercise*

The Princeton Plan recommends vigorous exercise *before* meals to
stimulate dietary-induced thermogenesis and reduce appetite. We also
recommend milder exercise—something as simple as a brisk walk—
after eating because studies indicate that this increases energy expenditure by 11 percent and also increases the amount of time the
metabolism remains elevated.

- **The greater your ratio of muscle mass to fat mass, the more
  calories you will burn all day long.** Muscle tissue is more
  metabolically active than fat. But building muscle does not
  mean that you need to enroll in an expensive health club and
  pump iron for hours. In chapter 14 we offer a number of
  strategies for increasing muscle in minutes a day, including a set
  of simple isometric exercises you can do at home. Building
  muscle will help you burn calories and will also help you
  streamline your body and improve muscle tone.

- **Alternating types of exercise *and* dietary composition can
  speed burning of fat stores.** It is often said that what we eat
  today provides the fuel for what we do tomorrow. Nowhere is
  this more important than in exercise.
  Intense, muscle-building exercises use stored carbohydrates, while sustained whole-body exercises eventually burn
  fat tissue directly. Thus, the Princeton Plan calls for muscle-
  building exercises on the day after the high-carbohydrate diet,
  to use the stored carbohydrates. On the next day, after the

low-carbohydrate diet, sustained exercise should be done to burn stored fat. (For more information, see pages 194–196 in Part III.)

5. The Princeton Plan Uses Specific Supplements to Enhance the Effects of All Other Parts of the Program

We recommend two types of supplements:

- **Vitamin and mineral supplements ensure optimum nutrition.** The Princeton Plan makes use of certain vitamin and mineral supplements for three reasons.

    First, any reduced-calorie diet is likely to be deficient in some micronutrients. According to the Food and Nutrition Board, a diet as low as 1800 to 2000 calories may be inadequate nutritionally. Since the Princeton Plan (and most other diets) is far lower in calories, it makes sense to take a daily multiple vitamin and mineral supplement to ensure that the minimum RDA is met for a variety of nutrients.

    Second, some micronutrients are needed in larger-than-normal amounts to stimulate metabolism, normalize insulin sensitivity, and increase thermogenesis.

    Third, exercise increases the need for some nutrients, such as the B-complex vitamins. In addition, water-soluble vitamins and minerals (for example, vitamin C and zinc) may be lost during exercise, through perspiration, and through the urine.

    Vitamins B_6 and B_3 are precursors to melatonin, a hormone that stimulates BAT, and to one of the "good" prostaglandins.

    Chromium, magnesium, and niacin, among other nutrients, are essential in normalizing insulin tolerance.

    Please note that none of the supplements we recommend is toxic at the levels recommended. Rather, we recommend supplying the body with appropriate amounts of all the nutrients it requires for optimum functioning of all its systems, including thermogenesis. See chapter 8 for complete details on which supplements to take and at what dosages.

- **The Princeton Plan Powdered Diet Drinks.** We have developed two special powdered diet drinks that may be used, if you wish, to ensure that you will be able to stick to the diet program more easily. One, the Princeton Plan LC formula, is for the low-calorie, low-carbohydrate day. The other, the Princeton Plan HC formula, is for the high-calorie, high-carbohydrate day. These drinks are optional and are not necessary for the Princeton Plan to be effective, but they may be substituted for one or more of the meals or snacks when you find it impossible to obtain the proper food (when traveling, too busy at work to get lunch or dinner, with the kids at special events, or during family emergencies).

To help you locate a store in your community that carries the Princeton Plan products, call (800) 635-4631.

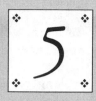

THE PRINCETON PLAN
PLUS

WE are very lucky to live at the end of the twentieth century. While it is true that the current American diet is essentially unhealthful, it is equally true that for the first time in history we have the nutritional and technological know-how to create a diet that can help our bodies function in the healthiest and most efficient way possible. We actually have the capability to create a better diet than the "natural" one on which our remote ancestors evolved.

The Princeton Plan provides such a diet. You are probably reading this book because you want to lose weight and keep it off, but the Princeton Plan can do far more for you than increase your thermogenesis. It is a comprehensive plan that can lead to improved overall health for a long and vigorous lifetime. To see why, let's take a closer look at the basic elements of the Plan.

FATS AND OILS

Although the Princeton Plan has a number of components, in many ways fat—the amount and type eaten—is the key to its success. As we saw in chapter 3, the essential fatty acids must be present in the diet in order for thermogenesis to take place. But the role of fats in maintaining the body goes much further, affecting virtually all metabolic processes.

The essential fatty acids belong to the group of fats known as **polyunsaturated**. This designation refers to molecular structure. Fats, like proteins and carbohydrates, consist of molecules made up primarily of carbon and hydrogen. (This is why your body is able to convert one type of nutrient to another—transforming carbohydrate, for example, into fat for storage.) In the case of fats, carbon atoms, the "spine" of a fat molecule, can attach to each other with either a single or a double bond. Where the bond is a double one, there is an electrochemical "space" available for a hydrogen atom to attach. The more such spaces that are actually occupied by hydrogen atoms, the more "saturated" that fat molecule is said to be. **Monounsaturated fats** contain one double bond between carbon atoms, while **polyunsaturated fats** have two or more double bonds between carbon atoms. **Hydrogenated fats** are unsaturated fats that, through chemical or heat processing, have had some of these spaces filled with hydrogen atoms; their properties thus resemble those of saturated fats.

None of this chemistry matters to us on a practical level; what does matter is the different ways in which these fats react in the body. Saturated fats, for example, have long been considered to be a prime cause of atherosclerosis, or "hardening of the arteries." Although recent studies cast doubt on this theory, the main problem with saturated fats is that like all fats they are calorie dense, and in the typical American diet they take up space that could otherwise be used by the essential fatty acids, which are so important in so many bodily processes. Remember, as we pointed out in chapter 3, that "you are what you eat" where fats are concerned; your body will make use of whatever fatty acids are contained in the cells, even if the particular fatty acid does not do the job as well or as efficiently as an essential fatty acid.

NATURAL AND UNNATURAL FATS

Unsaturated fats are further divided into another set of categories: **cis-** and **trans-**. The technical name for any polyunsaturated fatty acid usually has numbers in it and always starts with either the prefix *cis-* or *trans-*. **Cis-fatty acids** are the natural form, the one that is found in unspoiled seeds or leaves or roots. **Trans-fatty acids,** on the other hand, are polyunsaturated fats that have been chemically changed by such processing methods as heating at extremely high temperatures and treatment with harsh chemicals, to remove strong flavors or colors. The problem with trans-fatty acids is that although they retain all the same atoms as the natural cis- form, the molecule changes form in such a way that your body can't use it. Just as you can't wear a left shoe on your right foot, your body cannot use trans-fatty acids in its metabolic processes.

Saturated fats, on the other hand, can be used, but they compete with the essential fatty acids in certain metabolic processes. For example, if your body wants to make a certain prostaglandin that requires a molecule of an essential fatty acid, but in that organ system most of the fatty acids are saturated ones, the body is likely to use the saturated fatty acid, and the process your body is trying to complete will proceed inefficiently, or partially. Trans-fatty acids are far worse, however, because they compete with cis-fatty acids, *and* their very presence *blocks* essential-fatty-acid metabolism. Returning to the shoe analogy, it's as if the trans-fatty acids fill the shoe with putty, so that it cannot be used by a foot of any shape. Thus, if your body contains a great many trans-fatty acids, no matter how many essential fatty acids you ingest, your body will not be able to make full use of them. As a result, vital bodily processes will proceed sluggishly, if at all, and disease can develop.

The typical American diet, which, according to the Surgeon General, the American Heart Association, and other public health groups, is much too high in fat, gets 57 percent of that fat from commercially processed fats and oils. These can contain up to 60 percent or more chemically altered fatty acids and thus may contribute to many of the diseases of modern civilization, including cancer.

The good news is that the Princeton Plan, by emphasizing essential fatty acids and whole, unprocessed foods, greatly reduces the amount of saturated and trans-unsaturated fatty acids in the diet, allowing bodily functions to proceed efficiently. We also emphasize consumption of fish rich in omega-3 fish oils, which contain a metabolic by-product of one of the essential fatty acids in a form especially usable by the human body. We also recommend supplements, such as zinc and vitamin B_6, that work with the essential fatty acids in metabolic processes.

THE PROSTAGLANDIN CONNECTION

Bearing in mind again that essential fatty acids are precursors to prostaglandins (PGs), you can see how they are involved in virtually every biological process on a cellular level. Prostaglandins, which we discussed in chapter 3, are continually made and destroyed by the cells where they work. As we also mentioned earlier, they tend to work in pairs, with one PG causing, say, inflammation, while the other reduces it. Although all prostaglandins are "natural" and have important functions, they are divided into three general classes, called Series PG1, PG2, and PG3, of which two—PG1 and PG3—can broadly be considered "good" and one—PG2—"bad." The "bad" PG2-series prostaglandins are not really bad, but they are more active than the others and tend to cause undesirable effects, such as muscle cramping or inflammation.

Now, all prostaglandins are made from EFAs stored in cell membranes. *Which* fatty acids will be used depends entirely on the kinds of fats in your diet.

Unfortunately, if your diet is not rich in the essential fatty acids, or if there is too much saturated fat or highly processed unsaturated fat competing with the essential fatty acids, too many of the "bad" prostaglandins will be made relative to the "good" ones, leading to defective thermogenesis and to a number of undesirable health consequences. Too many of the wrong kinds of prostaglandins have been implicated in such maladies as arthritis, asthma, multiple sclerosis, heart disease, and even some forms of cancer.

By emphasizing large amounts of essential fatty acids, while limiting saturated and chemically processed unsaturated fats, the Princeton Plan helps to ensure that your body's cells have sufficient essential fatty acids to work with in their micromolecular processes.

CHOLESTEROL AND CARDIOVASCULAR DISEASE

You have no doubt read about cholesterol, a waxy substance usually found in the same foods that contain saturated fat. Cholesterol is a vital constituent of some hormones and is part of the structure of every animal cell wall. Our bodies are able to make as much cholesterol as we need, so we don't have to get it from the diet, but, unfortunately, many of us do get it that way, and in very large amounts.

For many years, medical thinking has held that excess cholesterol is primarily responsible for atherosclerosis, or coronary artery disease, in which **plaque**, which is composed of cholesterol and cellular debris, builds up on the inside walls of arteries, narrowing and ultimately blocking them.

More recent research indicates that the problem of plaque buildup results not so much from excess cholesterol as from excess fats, especially the wrong kinds of fats. To see how this works, let's take a closer look at how our body transports cholesterol and fat.

Neither cholesterol nor fat can be dissolved in water, so neither can move through the bloodstream without special preparation involving a class of molecules called **lipoproteins**. These are special proteins to which fat or cholesterol attaches in such a way that the "lipid" (fatty) part is on the inside. You can think of lipoproteins as little submarines, safely enclosing the insoluble substances for transport.

The two main classes of lipoproteins are high-density lipoproteins (HDLs) and low-density lipoproteins (LDLs). LDLs are the main transporter of cholesterol from the liver to the tissues (e.g., arteries). HDLs are the main transporter of cholesterol from the arteries to the liver. If your body has an excess of LDLs, more cholesterol will be deposited in the arteries, leading to buildups of cholesterol (e.g., arteriosclerosis).

While doctors still agree that it's important to have a low *total* cholesterol count, most experts now believe that far more important is your ratio of LDL to HDL. The higher the HDL, the better.

Enter now the ubiquitous essential fatty acids. Current research indicates that saturated fats raise blood cholesterol, while polyunsaturated fats lower it. But even more important, essential fatty acids change the *ratio* of LDL to HDL, raising the latter relative to the former.

Thus, the Princeton Plan works to lower cholesterol and increase the ratio of HDLs to LDLs in a number of ways.

1. Low total fat/low saturated fat. By emphasizing lean meats and nonfat dairy products, the Princeton Plan provides a diet much lower in saturated fat than the standard American diet; the

higher ratio of polyunsaturated fats helps to lower total cholesterol levels.

2. The high essential-fatty-acid content of the diet increases the
    ratio of HDL to LDL, resulting in less arterial buildup of
    cholesterol.

3. Low-cholesterol foods. Intake of excess cholesterol is primarily
    a problem for those who have a family history of high blood
    cholesterol. Since high cholesterol in foods generally goes
    hand in hand with high fat content, our Plan, by limiting fatty
    foods, also offers a lower cholesterol content than the standard
    American diet and many reducing diets as well.

4. In addition to the factors above, high fiber intake, exercise, and
    weight loss itself have all been proven to lower cholesterol. As
    a bonus, exercise increases the "good" HDL cholesterol.

STRONG BONES

Osteoporosis, a problem very common in postmenopausal women,
results when the bones lose calcium and become brittle, resulting in
easy breakage and such deformities as "dowager's hump."

The Princeton Plan helps prevent osteoporosis in four ways:

1. We include high-calcium foods and supplements, since most
    American women don't get enough calcium, even on a diet
    that is not calorie-restricted.

2. Studies indicate that a high-carbohydrate diet, like the Prince-
    ton Plan, can increase calcium absorption.

3. Regular weight-bearing exercise has been proven to increase
    bone density, *even in older women,* and to prevent further cal-
    cium loss.

4. Natural foods such as fruits contain boron, which is important
    in preventing osteoporosis.

DIABETES

We do not claim that the Princeton Plan can cure diabetes. But many adult-onset diabetics are able to control their insulin levels without medication by combining a healthful diet with exercise.

The principles of the Princeton Plan all combine to improve a diabetic condition as much as possible. Weight loss itself helps to normalize blood-sugar levels and decrease insulin resistance, a major problem for most adult-onset diabetics. A number of dietary strategies, discussed in chapter 4, also help control insulin resistance. In addition, many of the recommended supplements and micronutrients, including glucose tolerance factor (see page 236), can help to normalize carbohydrate metabolism in the body.

PREMATURE AGING

You may have heard of **free radicals**, which are implicated in degenerative changes in the body, contributing to a wide range of conditions from cancer to visible signs of aging. Although they may sound like subversive political cadres, free radicals are actually destructive molecules formed in the presence of oxygen that attack and break down healthy body structures, including the cell membranes, where many important biochemical processes take place.

There are always some free radicals present in the body; their amount and activity are greatly increased by such things as spoiled or rancid food, sunlight, pollution, and cigarette smoke. To prevent free-radical damage, your body makes use of antioxidant substances, such as vitamins E and C, beta-carotene, and selenium. By emphasizing adequate amounts of these nutrients in the diet, **the Princeton Plan can help you to minimize damage caused by free radicals, including premature aging.**

PMS AND CYSTIC BREAST DISEASE

PMS, or premenstrual syndrome, is said to affect the majority of women at some point in their reproductive lives. Symptoms range from the physical—bloating and cramping—to the psychological—irritability and depression. **The Princeton Plan can help alleviate PMS symptoms in a number of ways.** First, reducing sodium intake reduces bloating, while low-fat diets have been shown to reduce psychological symptoms. In addition, because of the rich supply of essential fatty acids and supplements, the Princeton Plan may reduce menstrual cramping, which is thought to be caused at least in part by "bad" prostaglandins. Our recommended supplements are essential for the formation of a prostaglandin (PGE1) known to alleviate menstrual distress.

Cystic breast disease, characterized by benign but often painful lumps in the breast, is considered by many experts to be largely caused by an unhealthful diet. Studies have shown that it, like menstrual disorders, usually improves on a low-fat, low-sodium diet that includes vitamin E and excludes methylxanthines. These substances, which include caffeine, theophylline, and theobromine, all of which are found in coffee, tea, and chocolate, can cause excessive stimulation of fibrous tissue.

DIGESTIVE DISORDERS

Common digestive complaints, ranging from indigestion to irritable bowel syndrome, often improve on a healthful diet. Quite obviously, **the Princeton Plan, by providing much more fiber than the standard American diet, increases bulk, thus reducing problems with constipation.** In addition, a high-fiber diet combined with exercise has been shown to speed intestinal transit time, the amount of time food spends in the intestines before being eliminated. Many experts believe that this reduces exposure of the bowels to toxic and possibly carcinogenic waste substances. In fact, too much fat and too little fiber are generally considered the two biggest dietary risk factors for colon, breast, and prostate cancer. Finally, emphasizing small, frequent meals that are not overly rich ensures that dieters will never feel bloated or stuffed after a meal, which often contributes to indigestion.

The Princeton Plan offers innumerable other health benefits. Because it consists of natural, nutrient-packed foods, you should never feel logy after a meal, and you may enjoy more energy than ever before. You may find that any recurrent skin problems clear up (a diet high in essential fatty acids is the ticket to a clear, healthy complexion). After you have been on the Princeton Plan for a few weeks, we think you will agree that it is not only the best reducing diet you have ever tried but also a natural and easy-to-follow regimen that you will want to continue through a long and healthy life.

PART II

THE PRINCETON
EATING PLAN

HOW MUCH SHOULD
YOU WEIGH?

Just as most diet plans ignore the biggest components of energy expenditure, and just as they focus on calories alone rather than whether those calories come from fat, carbohydrate, or protein, most diets also emphasize only weight loss. **The Princeton Plan is designed to lead to weight loss, but we are not interested in the loss of pounds so much as the loss of** *fat,* **which in terms of health is much more important.**

Most traditional diet books start with a discussion of how much you should weigh and usually include a variant of the Metropolitan Life height/weight charts, which present a range of "ideal" weights. These charts can serve as a useful guideline, but they are misleading in two respects. First, the range of weights they give represents only the weights at which there are fewest deaths, without taking other factors—like smoking—into account. Second, they completely ignore body composition—the percentage of your body that is made up of fat compared to lean tissue. It is possible to be at the "ideal" weight yet still possess far too much body fat. For example, a sedentary man who falls within the Metropolitan guidelines may look fine, but if he has too little muscle relative to his fat stores, he is actually in worse shape than a muscular football player who is 60 pounds "overweight" according to the charts. In fact, Mark Gastineau, the flamboyant former line-backer for the New York Jets, was once measured as having the lowest percentage of body fat among all pro football players—despite his weight of 275 pounds.

Although there have been few studies relating percentage of body fat to increased risk of disease, many researchers are coming to believe that it may be even more important than overall weight in determining health. The location of fat on your body is important, too; according to the Human Nutrition Research Center of the USDA, people who deposit fat primarily in the abdomen and around the waist are at greater risk for heart disease, diabetes, and hypertension than those whose fat stores are largely in the hips and thighs.

The Princeton Plan attacks excess fat on two fronts: First, as we pointed out in Part I, numerous studies confirm that the lower in fat your diet, the less likely you are to deposit excess calories as body fat. Second, exercise burns not only calories but fat, using it for fuel (for details, see chapter 13).

How much body fat is healthy? In general, experts consider 18 to 25 percent fat to be normal for healthy women, although the lower figure is more desirable. For men, 10 to 18 percent body fat is consid-ered the normal range (men naturally have more muscle than women do). Trained athletes may possess less than 10 percent body fat, but that is an ideal hard to attain and not necessary for most people. In fact, women with such low fat levels usually stop menstruating and may find it difficult or impossible to conceive.

A scientific determination of body-fat percentage involves immer-sion in a special tank of water called a *hydrodensitometer,* but you can easily get an idea of your own percentage of body fat by performing the following simple test: Lie on your back on a flat surface. Now, place a ruler along your body, with one end resting on your breastbone and the other on your abdomen. If the ruler slants downward, toward your abdomen, you are probably not carrying too much fat. If it slants upward, however, you need to lose weight—and fat.

Physiologist Jack H. Wilmore, in *Sensible Fitness* (Champaign, IL: Leisure Press, 1986), offers the following test, which requires only a tape measure:

For women, measure your hips at the widest point. Then, using the women's chart on page 47 and a straight edge, connect the measure-ment of hip girth to the measurement of your height, in inches. The point at which it crosses the "percent fat" scale is a rough estimate of your body-fat percentage.

For men, measure your waist at belly-button level. Then, using the men's chart and a straight edge, connect the waist measurement to the measure of your weight. The point at which it crosses the "percent fat" scale is a rough estimate of your body-fat percentage.

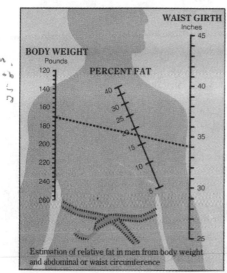

Estimation of relative fat in men from body weight and abdominal or waist circumference

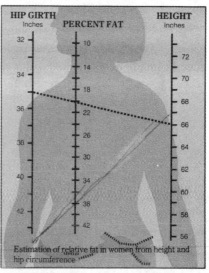

Estimation of relative fat in women from height and hip circumference

38%!

Charts reprinted with permission of *American Health* (July 1987).

BEWARE OF DIETING

It may seem strange, in a diet book, to offer a warning about dieting, but we don't want you to begin our plan frivolously or half-heartedly. Overwhelming evidence now indicates that yo-yo dieting—repeatedly losing and regaining weight—is very unhealthful and can increase the risk of heart disease. Therefore, we urge you not to begin this diet until you are certain that you want to lose weight and keep it off by a *permanent* change in your eating habits and life-style.

Second, before you begin, be sure that you have a realistic idea of the amount of weight you need to lose. Many overweight people have an unrealistic body image, and even when they have lost a great deal of weight still see themselves as "fat." This misperception can sometimes lead to eating disorders such as bulimia and anorexia.

One way to gauge your ideal weight is to aim for approximately the weight you had when you were twenty, unless you were very overweight then. Alternatively, consult your doctor, or use a standard height-weight chart as a rough guideline. Bear in mind, too, that not everyone can be as svelte as the models in magazine ads; take a look at close family members—you may be a big-boned person that no amount of dieting is going to make skinny.

Remember that you are adopting the Princeton Plan as part of a long-term, positive change in your life and that as long as you continue to follow our guidelines, treating your body to complete nutrition, you should steadily replace fat with lean muscle tissue and move ever closer to your goal of vibrant health and a sensible body weight.

COOKING THE
PRINCETON WAY

ONE great advantage of the Princeton Plan is that it can be adapted to all kinds of cookery. If you are a no-fuss, no-bother cook who doesn't want to spend a lot of time in the kitchen, you will find that the Plan easily lends itself to the use of convenience foods and prepare-ahead dishes.

On the other hand, if you enjoy cooking, the Plan is perfect for you, because in emphasizing whole-food ingredients and herbs and spices, it offers wide scope for culinary creativity. Once you get used to cooking the Princeton way, the variety of foods you can prepare is virtually endless and includes healthful adaptations of "gourmet" recipes as well as favorite family treats.

Although experienced cooks will probably be able to begin cooking immediately, you may find it helpful to read through the following pages for guidelines and tips on cooking foods the Princeton way.

LOWER-FAT COOKING

Probably the biggest difference between cooking on the Princeton Plan and the way you are accustomed to preparing meals is our emphasis on reducing fats, especially animal fats and unnatural, processed oils, and our elimination of traditional oil-frying.

Although we do not offer equivalents for such foods as deep-fried French fries (although "oven-fried" chips are delicious), you will be able to prepare healthful versions of nearly any favorite dish. In fact, after you have been eating on the Princeton Plan for a few weeks, you will probably find that many of your former high-fat favorites don't taste good any more, or, as one woman we know who switched to lower-fat eating put it, "All I can taste now is the grease."

Adapting to lower-fat menus is not difficult, as long as you keep in mind a few basic guidelines. The first is that there are a limited number of foods you must simply learn to avoid, starting with all deep-fried and commercially fried foods. Not only are these foods high in overall fat (as much as 60 percent of the calories in French fries comes from fat!); much of that fat is the unnatural kind that interferes with essential-fatty-acid metabolism.

You must also learn to say no to such calorie-dense but nutrition-poor items as ice cream, margarine, and gravies. This in no way means, however, that from now on all of the food you ingest will be dry, tasteless, or textureless. Quite the opposite! For one thing, the fats you will use—natural, unprocessed seed and nut oils—are in themselves tasty, adding delicate flavors and overtones to all foods they are combined with. In addition, there are innumerable ways to prepare food without using animal fats or processed oils, and many of these techniques, in addition to being healthful, also result in a better texture, appearance, and flavor than traditional oil-frying.

- **Sautéing in PAM.** PAM is a commercial product made of lecithin, a natural component of vegetable oils. Though not a fat itself, PAM prevents food from sticking as it is cooked and thus can be used in place of oil or fat for "frying" and "sautéing." A spray of PAM instead of 2 teaspoons of oil eliminates 80 calories, yet foods prepared this way have a flavor and texture similar to those that are fried in oil.

    To use PAM, spray it on the surface of a pan, heat to

cooking temperature, then add food and cook just as if you were sautéing. (You can even "stir-fry" with PAM for Oriental dishes).

PAM can also be used on baking dishes to prevent casseroles or baked goods from sticking.

Please note that we do not emphasize the use of PAM in our recipe section, because the essential fatty acids contained in our recommended cooking oils will help speed weight loss. Once you have achieved your weight-loss goal, however, and are eating higher-calorie meals, cooking with PAM can be an excellent way to cut down on excess calories.

- **Steaming.** Steaming is one of the easiest and most healthful ways to prepare a variety of foods, especially vegetables. Steamed foods retain far more vitamins and minerals than foods that are boiled.

  Although it is not absolutely necessary, it is helpful to get a collapsible steamer basket, which you can find in hardware stores and houseware departments for under $10. You can also use a wire rack or slotted metal trivet, but these do not adapt to any size of pan, as the collapsible basket does.

  To steam vegetables, put ½ to 1 inch of water in the bottom of a saucepan with a tight-fitting lid. Insert the steamer basket, bring the water to a boil, then put the washed and cut vegetables in the steamer. Cover the pan tightly, and turn down the heat.

  Steaming times will vary depending on the particular food being cooked, but in general, vegetables will take as much or less time than if boiled. For example (and depending on how well-done you like your vegetables), zucchini takes about 5 minutes, broccoli 6 to 9 minutes, and potatoes 20 to 25 minutes.

  You can steam several vegetables at the same time, simply adding the quicker-cooking ones later.

- **Broiling.** Another healthful way to prepare foods, especially meat and fish, is broiling in an oven broiler or toaster oven. To prevent sticking, first spray the broiler pan with PAM, then heat. Add the meat or fish, and sprinkle with lemon or baste with nonfat marinade or marinade made with unprocessed oils containing essential fatty acids.

- **Baking or roasting.** You can bake or roast a wide variety of foods, including fish, meat, poultry, vegetables, casseroles, and even snacks such as thin potato slices or pumpkin and squash seeds. Use PAM instead of oil on the cooking pan, and for foods that might become dry, baste with tomato juice, lemon, or any low-fat marinade.

- **Microwaving.** Current estimates predict that more than 75 percent of American families will own a microwave oven by 1990, which means that few people will have an excuse to avoid healthful cooking and eating. A microwave saves time in the kitchen—most dishes cook in one-fourth the traditional cooking time—and can easily be adapted to low-fat cooking. Microwave ovens are especially good for cooking foods with a high water content, such as fish, chicken, and most vegetables. Learning to use a microwave oven is not difficult, as long as you follow a few simple guidelines. First, foods should be cooked in fairly small chunks—1-inch sections of broccoli work better than a whole stalk. Second, potatoes, squash, and other produce should be pierced with a fork before baking to prevent an "explosion." Finally, to prevent cold spots, rotate or stir food halfway through the cooking time.

  When preparing a large casserole, undercook it by 10 minutes, then divide it into several "Princeton-sized" portions and freeze. When you feel like "fast food," open one of these homemade TV dinners and microwave.

SUBSTITUTES FOR FATTY FOODS

Once you become conscious of the empty calories in your accustomed diet, you will discover many ways in which you can easily eliminate fat without sacrificing flavor. There are a number of healthful foods that can be substituted for high-fat foods. The list below is by no means exhaustive, but it will give you an idea of the types of creative substitutions you can make.

- **Low-fat yogurt.** Use low-fat yogurt in place of mayonnaise, sour cream, and cream. In many recipes, such as those for party dips, you may not notice a difference between the healthful dip and the fatty variety. In other recipes, such as tuna salad, yogurt is good for moistening the tuna mixture but does not confer quite the same texture as mayonnaise. For a thicker-textured yogurt, drain it through cheesecloth, discarding the liquid whey and retaining the "yogurt cheese" in the cheesecloth (special funnels for this purpose may be found at housewares stores or natural-food stores). This thickened yogurt is also excellent on baked potatoes.

Mixed with fresh chopped dill, yogurt makes a refreshing salad dressing; blended with mustard, a zesty sauce for vegetables; and seasoned with herbs or chili powder, a delicious dip. When cooking with yogurt (as in beef Stroganoff, for example), mix each cup of yogurt with 1 tablespoon of flour or 1 teaspoon of cornstarch to keep it from separating.

- **Hoop cheese.** This very low-fat product, also known as **whey cheese,** was described (unfairly, we think) by a prominent New York City cheese merchant as "a unique amalgam of library paste and cardboard." Although hoop cheese is definitely *not* a strong-flavored cheese, it has a subtle, creamy taste and texture that make it ideal as a substitute for cream cheese or sour cream in some recipes.

  Alone or mixed with herbs, hoop cheese makes an ideal spread on bread and crackers. In cooking, add it to pasta dishes that call for cream or sour cream.

- **Butter Buds.** This is a commercial flavoring that tastes approximately like butter. It comes in two forms: powdered and granular. The powder contains no fat, while the granulated variety contains some partially hydrogenated fat. Both products are high in sodium and should be used very sparingly.

  Despite its health drawbacks, the familiar taste of Butter Buds can ease the transition between standard American eating and the Princeton Plan. To use it, sprinkle the granules on hot, moist foods (such as cooked vegetables, hot cereals, or pasta) and mix well. The powdered form can also be sprinkled on, or it can be mixed with hot water and then drizzled on baked potatoes or other food. Mixed with skim milk and flour or corn starch, it can also be used to make an acceptable white sauce. Butter Buds cannot be used for frying, and its texture is nothing like that of butter.

- **Condensed skim milk.** If you find regular skim milk too "light" for your coffee, try the canned, condensed version, which contains no fat but has a satisfyingly "thick" feel. This product can also be used in most recipes that call for whole milk, half-and-half, or cream.

- **Sunflower seeds and pumpkin seeds.** Use these instead of fatty croutons for a "crunch" in salads or for snacking. Although sunflower seeds, like all nuts and seeds, are high in fat, approximately two-thirds of that is polyunsaturated fat, including the essential fatty acid linoleic acid. For added flavor, try toasting the seeds by spreading them on a cookie sheet and placing in a 350°F oven for about 20 minutes.

GETTING OUT THE SALT

Cutting back on salt is one of the easiest healthful dietary changes you can make, and it can be done gradually or all at once. If you switch to low-salt eating "cold turkey," you will probably find that most foods taste bland for a few days to a week. But once you have kicked your sodium habit you will discover a new world of subtle flavors you hadn't dreamed existed—because all along what you had been tasting was the salt.

When cooking pasta, it is not necessary to add either salt or oil to the water. To keep the pasta from sticking together, stir vigorously as you add the dried product to boiling water. Continue to stir from time to time once the water has returned to a boil. If your pasta sauce is well seasoned, it should not require any salt at all, but if you feel you must have some, add it—sparingly—at the table.

As you become accustomed to low-salt cooking, we recommend experimenting with different seasonings and condiments. Below is a partial list of some of the items you may want to add for extra flavor.

- **Lemon juice.** Fresh-squeezed lemon juice is delicious on vegetables, salads, fruit, rice, potatoes, and many other dishes, adding an extra piquancy but no sodium or fat.

- **Red-pepper flakes.** These flakes, which contain the thermogenic substance capsaicin, put extra zip into any dish. They are especially good judiciously sprinkled on salads, in soups, and in tomato sauces.

- **Salsa.** Salsa, a key ingredient in many Mexican foods, also lends itself to a variety of other cuisines: It is good alone as a dip, or mixed with bland foods such as rice and beans. Because one of the main ingredients of salsa is chile pepper, it is also high in capsaicin while low in fat and calories.

  You can buy salsa ready-made in a variety of strengths ranging from just tangy to three-alarm, but check commercial brands for sodium content. It is easy to make your own salsa; for a recipe, see page 107.

- **Mustard.** Bottled mustard is delicious brushed as a condiment on broiled fish or chicken. For extra zip and eye appeal, add a sprinkle of paprika, red pepper, or parsley.

- **Herbs and spices.** Both fresh and dried, bottled herbs add flavor without adding fat or sodium. In addition to red and black pepper there is a whole world of spices that can be used individually or in combination to add interest to foods. If you are not used to cooking with herbs and spices, go easy at first, adding just enough to impart a subtle flavor. But don't be afraid to experiment. Indian cookbooks usually offer dozens of examples of marinades and seasonings, some containing a half dozen or more different herbs and spices.

  Although the following list is far from exhaustive, it gives some idea of the food-and-seasoning combos that seem to go together naturally.

  Meat: allspice, garlic, marjoram, thyme
  Poultry: garlic, marjoram, rosemary, tarragon, sage
  Fish: chives, dill, tarragon
  Tomatoes: basil, red pepper, tarragon
  Green vegetables: caraway, "curry" powder, dill, marjoram, rosemary

- **Lawry's Salt-Free Natural-Choice Seasonings.** These commercial products, made without sugar or preservatives, blend herbs and spices in three convenient "shakes"—one for vegetables and salads, one for meat, and one for chicken and fish.

- **McCormick's Parsley Patch** herb and spice blends. These additive-free seasonings blend herbs and spices in several tasty shakes. Especially versatile is "It's a Dilly," a dill-based shake good in salad dressings and soups, or mixed with yogurt as a dip.

You can also make your own substitute shakes with the following recipes:

Sesame Salt

Grind toasted sesame seeds coarsely. Add 1 part salt to 8 parts seeds. You can toast your own seeds by spreading them on a baking sheet and placing in a 350°F oven for 15 to 20 minutes.

Mary Conover's Substitute Salt

Put the following in blender and blend until fine: ¼ teaspoon dillweed, ¼ teaspoon marjoram, 1 teaspoon parsley, 1 teaspoon whole celery seed, 1¼ teaspoons garlic powder, 4½ teaspoons onion powder.

Yield: about 3 tablespoons

The following two shakes are recommended by Frances Sheridan Goulart, a well-known nutrition writer:

Lemon Salt

Grind the following in a spice mill, blender, or mortar: 1 teaspoon dried lemon or lime peel, 2 tablespoons black peppercorns, 1 teaspoon finely grated dried gingerroot (or ½ teaspoon nutmeg), 2 teaspoons powdered seaweed, such as kelp or dulse (optional), 1 teaspoon fennel or anise seed.

Yield: approximately ¼ cup

Pâté Maison "Salt"

Grind the following in a blender or spice grinder: ½ teaspoon *each* powdered bay leaves, cloves, nutmeg, paprika, and thyme; ¾ teaspoon *each* basil, cinnamon, oregano, sage, and savory; ¼ cup white peppercorns.

This traditional French spice mix can be used with salads or vegetables, sprinkled over chips, and used as a flavoring in pot roasts and stews.

Yield: 6 tablespoons

TIPS FOR HEALTHFUL COOKING AND ADAPTING RECIPES

As you become used to low-fat, low-salt cookery, you will be able to adapt recipes almost automatically. In the meantime, here are some tips to help you get maximum flavor and nutrition into every meal.

- Go easy on meat and cheese. You have probably heard that in Oriental cooking, which in its traditional form is a very healthful, low-fat cuisine, meat is used as a "condiment," rather than as the basis of a meal. In the Princeton Plan we adopt that approach and extend it to cheese as well. As you will see, our recipes use very small amounts of cheese and emphasize the low-fat varieties such as cottage cheese and hoop cheese. Most hard cheeses should be used very sparingly, because they are extremely high in saturated fat. Luckily, most hard cheeses are also strongly flavored, so it doesn't take much to add a cheesy taste to most dishes.

- When preparing chicken, remove the skin *before* cooking (most of the fat is in the skin). Removing the skin after cooking also eliminates fat, but not as much.

  Likewise, remove all visible fat from beef and other red meat *before* cooking. A Texas study proved that this can save up to 40 calories per 8-ounce portion, compared to removing the fat after cooking. Choose the lowest-fat grades of beef (which are usually the cheapest, as well): For example, when making beef Stroganoff, use round steak in place of sirloin.

✳ *Note:* To guard against salmonella poisoning, treat raw chicken (and fish) with caution. Don't place it on a board or platter you will be using later, and wash all utensils that come in contact with it (and your hands, too!) in hot, soapy water.

- When cooking chicken or beef for stock, or when making a meat-based stew or soup, refrigerate the broth overnight. In the morning, remove the congealed fat.

- Beware of many "natural foods" and "vegetarian" cookbooks. Unless the authors state that their recipes are low-fat, chances are they are high in unnecessary fat, literally "larded" with cheese and oils.

- If you buy commercial peanut butter, get the "old-fashioned," unsalted variety and pour off the extra oil instead of mixing it into the spread.

- When baking, remember that two egg whites can usually be used in place of one whole egg, eliminating nearly all the fat and all the cholesterol, and retaining most of the protein. You can also make omelets using only the egg white, or using two or more egg whites for each egg yolk (see recipes, chapter 9).

- Although we recommend cutting back on sweets as much as possible, to help break the sweet-addiction cycle, sweeteners are often called for in our recipes. In many cases, you can substitute frozen juice concentrates for sugar; frozen apple juice is especially good.

HEALTHFUL DRESSINGS FOR PASTA AND SALADS

Remember that all oils *are not* forbidden on the Princeton Plan, because the essential fatty acids found in unprocessed oils stimulate thermogenesis. The Plan offers generous amounts of these oils in uncooked dressings.

Look in health-food stores for oils labeled *cold-pressed, mechanical process, unrefined, virgin,* or *extra virgin.* These oils are richer in color than processed oils and smell and taste like the seed, nut, or grain from which they originated. Oils may be blended to create distinctive tastes.

The oils that are richest in essential fatty acids include linseed (flax), canola (rapeseed), corn, safflower, sesame, soybean, and sunflower oils (see the chart on page 60 for a complete breakdown). Olive oil is also good for a change of pace; its monounsaturated fatty acids block the synthesis of arachidonic acid. (**Arachidonic acid** is a fatty acid important in many biological processes, but it is widely available in the diet and can also be made from the essential fatty acid linoleic acid. Excessive arachidonic acid relative to other fatty acids results in production of the "harmful" prostaglandin series and consequent health problems.)

Remember that fresh, unprocessed oils are very fragile and must be refrigerated to prevent rancidity. Rancid oil is extremely toxic, and, unfortunately, it cannot be detected by smell or taste until it has been rancid for some time. To make certain that the oils you use are fresh, become acquainted with the odor and flavor of a variety of fresh oils. Get used to smelling them as soon as you open them. Each oil's characteristic odor will become familiar in time, and soon you'll be able to tell one from another blindfolded. Once again, remember that unprocessed oils should smell and taste like the seed, nut, or grain from which they originated. If you notice any unpleasant, sour, bitter, or rank odor or taste, that is a warning that the oil has become rancid; discard it immediately.

To create your own dressings, mix vinegar or lemon juice with the oil of your choice, in a 1:2 ratio (one part vinegar or lemon to two parts oil). Then add seasonings, to taste. The usual seasonings include garlic, mustard, chopped green herbs (such as parsley and chives), and tarragon or basil. For a really special dressing, use herbed or fruit vinegars. If you want more dressing than the amount allowed in a recipe, simply add water to expand.

For more detailed instructions on preparing dressings, see the recipes in chapter 9.

% FATTY-ACID CONTENT OF OILS

Oil	Cis-linoleic (Omega-6 Fatty Acid) C-LA	Alpha-linolenic (Omega-3 Fatty Acid) ALA	Mono-unsatu-rated	Poly-unsatu-rated	Satu-rated
Almond	24		68	24	8
Apricot kernel*	29		60	29	6
Coconut	2		6	2	91
Corn	56	1	28	57	14
Cottonseed	52	2	19	54	27
Linseed (flax)	15	53	21	68	11
Olive					
European	9	1	75	10	15
Tunisian	19	1	61	20	19
Palm	10	1	37	11	52
Palm-kernel	3		14	3	83
Peanut	29	1	50	30	20
Rapeseed* (Canola)	22	11	56	33	7
Safflower	74	1	13	75	11
Sesame	42	2	41	43	16
Soybean	52	9	23	61	16
Sunflower	65		23	65	12
Walnut	60	13	19	73	9

Source: Geigy Scientific Tables, vol. 1, edited by C. Lentner (CIBA-GEIGY, 1981), 264.

Source: Consumer and Food Economics Institute, *Composition of Foods: Fats and Oils,* Agriculture Handbook No. 8-4, United States Department of Agriculture, Science and Education Administration. Revised June 1979.

Note: The total monounsaturated, polyunsaturated, and saturated percentages do not always add up to exactly 100 percent because of rounding-off errors or errors in the actual analysis.

CHOOSING FRESH FISH

There is no doubt that most fish, with its rich supply of essential fatty acids (see chart on page 62), is a healthy choice. Fear of pollutants does not mean that consumers need to swear off fish. Much of the seafood sold at supermarkets and other reputable retailers is caught deep at sea where the water is clean.

USING CONVENIENCE FOODS

It is unfortunate that we cannot yet go to a supermarket and buy a wide variety of healthful dishes ready-made. All supermarkets, however, stock a number of convenience foods that fit the Princeton Plan guidelines.

The most important thing to bear in mind when you are shopping for convenience foods is to *read the labels,* checking sodium, sugar, and fat content.

Labeling information is provided in two parts: a list of ingredients, which is required on most packaged foods, and nutritional labeling, which is optional. Of the two, the nutritional labeling is the more useful, as it provides the actual content of key nutrients.

Sodium content is listed on labels in grams or milligrams per serving. Our goal is to keep total daily sodium intake under 2000 mg. (2 grams). Once you begin reading labels, you may be shocked to discover the sodium content of some foods. A popular brand of soup, for example, offers three versions of chicken noodle soup—low-sodium, regular, and chunky. Comparing the nutritional content reveals that these soups contain, per serving, 85, 910, and 1140 mg. of sodium respectively. A single bowl of the chunky variety would account for more than 50 percent of your entire day's sodium allowance!

Checking labels for fat content is somewhat trickier, because you must keep in mind not only the *amount* of fat but also the *kind* of fat used. Beware of labels that proclaim "All vegetable oil—no cholesterol." Many products so labeled contain tropical oils, such as palm and coconut oil, both of which are highly saturated. Remember, too, that many commercial products, including most baked goods and desserts,

FISH AND SHELLFISH SOURCES OF
OMEGA-3 FATTY ACIDS

Grams of Omega-3 Fatty Acids Per 3.5-ounce
Portion*

Chinook salmon (canned)	3.0
Other salmon	1.0–1.9
Norway sardines	2.9
Mackerel (Atlantic)	2.2–2.6
Lake trout	2.0
Herring (Atlantic)	1.7
Albacore tuna	1.5–1.7
Eel	1.6
Sablefish	1.4
Anchovy	1.4
Bluefish	1.2
Rainbow trout	1.1
Squid	.9
Halibut	.5–.9
Oyster	.8
Striped bass	.6
Catfish	.6
King crab	.6
Ocean perch	.5
Blue crab (canned)	.5
Shrimp	.4
Flounder	.3
Haddock	.2
Lobster	.2
Scallops	.2
Red snapper	.2
Swordfish	.2

*For comparison: One typical capsule of fish oil contains .3 grams of omega-3 fatty acids.

are made with highly processed, unnatural oils that interfere with essential-fatty-acid metabolism.

A quick way to determine the fat content of a prepared food is to see where, on the list of ingredients, fat appears. Manufacturers are required by law to list ingredients by weight, in descending order. Thus, if fat is one of the first three or four items on the list, chances are it is a high-fat product.

If a product provides nutritional labeling, you can determine its fat content more exactly. To do this, you need two items on the label: total calories and grams of fat. One gram of fat equals 9 calories. Our goal is to keep the percentage of fat at 25 percent or less. To determine the *percentage* of fat in a product, multiply the number of fat grams by 9, and divide the total by the total number of calories. Thus, in a prepared split-pea soup that contains 80 calories per serving, with 1 gram of fat, the formula is $9 \times 1 = 9$; divided by 80, giving us a little more than 11 percent fat, a very healthful total.

Checking sugar content is the trickiest of all, because sugar may be listed under a variety of names: sugar, sucrose, glucose, maltose, dextrose, corn sugar, corn syrup, levulose, sorbitol, fructose, lactose, galactose, mannitol, honey, high-fructose corn syrup, molasses, maple syrup, turbinado, and hexitol. If one or more of the above is listed in the top three or four ingredients, that product contains too much sugar. If sugar appears as the fifth or sixth item, it is probably acceptable. Don't assume that just because a food doesn't taste sweet it is low in sugar—added sugar appears in many products where you wouldn't expect it, in everything from high-fiber cereals to stewed tomatoes.

When you can, avoid products that do not provide nutritional labeling. Fortunately, increasing numbers of manufacturers are listing this valuable information in response to consumer demand.

Finally, although there are a number of very healthful convenience products offered in health-food stores, many of these items are just as high in fat and sodium as those found in supermarkets (and more expensive, too). Remember to read the label!

The following convenience foods can generally be used within the Princeton Plan guidelines.

- **Canned beans.** These can be a real time-saver in the kitchen, since most dried beans take from one to several hours to cook from scratch. Be aware, however, that most commercial brands of beans contain high levels of sodium; rinsing the beans in a colander will get rid of most of this excess salt without washing away significant amounts of other nutrients. (For instructions on cooking beans from scratch, see pages 108–110.)

- **Canned tomatoes and tomato sauce.** These, like beans, generally contain too much salt, but a few companies have begun to come out with low-sodium varieties. Particularly in the winter, when fresh tomatoes are scarce, these products can streamline meal preparation.

- **Canned spaghetti sauce.** Most commercial brands of spaghetti sauce contain too much fat, salt, and sugar (read the labels!). A number of health-food store brands, including Pritikin and Enrico's, are acceptably low in all these ingredients, although both are much more expensive than supermarket brands.

- **Canned soups.** Again, there is far too much fat, salt, and sugar in most commercial soups, although more reduced-salt varieties are beginning to appear. Health-food brands vary from variety to variety as well as among brands, although all Pritikin soups contain no fat and are low in sodium (and high in cost).

  When you are too busy to make a soup stock of your own (or if you never do it), a good bet is to buy a can of commercial low-salt chicken broth and refrigerate it for at least two hours. When you open the can you will find that all of the fat has congealed at the top and can easily be discarded. (The surprisingly large amount of sticky yellow fat provides a vivid demonstration of the "hidden" fats found in many canned products.)

- **Canned fish.** Always buy tuna packed in spring water (get the reduced-sodium kind if you can find it); rinsing will get rid of much of the excess salt.

  Red and pink salmon are a delicious, if somewhat expensive, source of a number of nutrients. They supply generous amounts of calcium. Use them in addition to tuna for sandwiches and salads.

  Sardines packed in sild oil—the natural oil of the sardine— are a rich, inexpensive source of the fish-derived omega-3 oils. As with salmon, eat the bones in canned fish for extra calcium.

- **Instant brown rice.** Although not as "chewy" as the long-cooking variety, instant brown rice is virtually as nutritious and takes only 12 minutes to cook, 5 minutes less than regular white rice.

- **Low-calorie salad dressings and mayonnaise.** When choosing reduced-calorie bottled dressings or mayonnaise, check the label to make sure the product contains no sugar, hydrogenated oil, palm oil, or coconut oil.

THE TWO-WEEK PRINCETON EATING PLAN

Now you are ready to begin the Princeton Eating Plan. Remember that unlike traditional diets, it has three essential elements:

1. whole foods and selected supplements to ensure that all nutritional needs are met;

2. generous amounts of essential fatty acids for production of "good" prostaglandins and thermogenesis;

3. alternating low-carbohydrate, low-calorie days and high-carbohydrate, high-calorie days for metabolic stimulation.

For convenience, you may want to think of the high-carbohydrate days as vegetarian days; because of the generous amount of protein in the grains and beans, only a token amount of meat should be eaten on those days.

In the next pages you will find everything you need to follow the Princeton Eating Plan. (For details on combining it with the Princeton

Exercise Plan, see Part III.) In this chapter, we provide fourteen full days of menus for both men and women, a chart of daily supplements, a list of "free foods" that you may eat in unlimited quantities, a list of all allowed beverages, and details on how to use the Princeton Plan LC and HC powdered diet drinks.

For best results, please follow these menus as exactly as possible. While it won't hurt to switch two similar meals occasionally (say, eating the Day 4 high-carbohydrate breakfast on Day 2 or Day 6), you must *never* switch two meals of different types (for example, eating a low-carbohydrate dinner instead of a high-carbohydrate dinner). Furthermore, remember that we designed the alternating menus to maximize thermogenesis and thus speed weight loss: Each food item listed for each day works with all of that day's other foods to increase metabolism while providing all the micronutrients necessary for good health and weight loss.

If you find it difficult to deal with so much variety in your diet (and we know some people do), turn to chapter 11, "The Six-Day Rotation Plan," which provides a week of predictable menus while still alternating low-carbohydrate, low-calorie days with high-carbohydrate, high-calorie days and providing all needed nutrition.

Chapter 9 contains recipes for all dishes in capital letters in the menus. For simpler recipes, such as salads and sandwiches, the menus instruct you to "combine for a salad/sandwich."

Whenever the word *dressing* is listed in a menu or recipe, choose any dressing on pages 104–106, or create your own, as described on page 59. Remember that the fresh oils used in these dressings are essential for thermogenesis and weight loss, so do *not* choose a low-calorie or no-calorie dressing where dressing is *specified.*

When preparing meals, bear in mind that the *size* of each portion is important. It may help to use a food scale or a postage scale until you have learned the approximate sizes of given portions of food (for instance, 4 ounces of meat is about the size of a deck of cards; a 3-ounce potato is about the size of an egg, and so on).

After you have followed the Two-Week Eating Plan for several weeks, you will probably want to begin planning your own meals. To do so, turn to chapter 10, "Your Personal Eating Plan." Once you have become familiar with the Exchange Lists in that section, you can also make modifications to the menus in this basic plan.

Finally, for convenience, especially if you travel or eat out frequently, in chapter 11 we offer a Six-Day Rotation Plan, in which meals and snacks are predictable from day to day and any given meal (e.g., a low-carbohydrate breakfast) can be exchanged with any other *equivalent* meal during the week.

Instead of the above, you can always use the Princeton Plan LC or HC powdered diet drinks. These are two different formulas specially created according to the specifications for the Princeton Plan LC and HC days. The LC formula contains 200 calories per packet and the correct proportions of carbohydrate, protein, and fat to be used on the low-calorie, low-carbohydrate day. The HC formula contains 300 calories per packet and the correct proportions of carbohydrate, protein, and fat to be used on the high-calorie, high-carbohydrate day.

The appropriate formula may be substituted for any one of your meals or snacks. For instance, if you wake up late on a day when you are supposed to have your high-carbohydrate breakfast but will miss the train if you eat, you can grab a packet of the HC formula and take it to work with you. The packets are made to be mixed with water and stirred or blended in a blender. If you have to miss a dinner meal on the low-carbohydrate day, you can use two packets of the powder for the LC day, giving you 400 calories. And finally, if you need a snack and can't get one, you can use one half of the packet for the appropriate day.

We emphasize that real food is to be eaten whenever possible. But we also realize that you are only human and sometimes circumstances prevent you from carrying out your best intentions. Rather than go off the diet and eat incorrectly for one or several meals, please remember you can use the "quick fix" formula.

Do not, however, use just the powdered formula for the entire day. This is very dangerous and anyone doing such a thing must be monitored by a physician so that electrolyte imbalances and cardiac problems do not occur. If the powdered formula is used for breakfast, lunch, and snacks, the dinner meal must consist of the prescribed **foods** for that day.

To help you locate a store in your area that carries the Princeton Plan LC and Princeton Plan HC powdered drinks, call (800) 635-4631.

Note: The menus for men alternate between 1200 and 1700 calories, for an average of roughly 1500 calories, because studies show that this is the calorie level at which most men lose weight. Likewise, the women's menus average 1200 calories, for the same reason. If you find that you need fewer or more calories to achieve your goals, turn to Appendix A for complete details on modifying the basic diet.

MEN'S 1500-CALORIE ALTERNATING PLAN

The following menus provide three meals and three snacks a day for fourteen days. The reducing plan consists of a diet that averages roughly 1500 calories, alternating between 1200- and 1700-calorie days.

❖   ❖

Day 1, Men
Low-calorie, low-carbohydrate
1200 calories

Breakfast

French Toast with Applesauce (see page 111)

Snack

1 cup skim milk

Lunch

Tuna Salad (see page 116)
Lettuce
1 large tomato, sliced

Snack

1 pita (6 inches across)
Salad greens: endive, escarole, spinach, lettuce, romaine

Dinner

4 ounces (cooked weight) lean broiled steak (see page 120)
1 small (3-ounce) baked potato
Dilled Zucchini (see page 120)

Snack

15 grapes (red or green)

❖   ❖

Day 2, Men
High-calorie, high-carbohydrate
1700 calories

Breakfast

1 cup concentrated, uncooked bran cereal (containing little or no sugar, such as Kellogg's All Bran with extra fiber)
1 cup skim milk (use desired amount on cereal and drink the rest)

Snack

1/2 medium grapefruit or 3/4 cup grapefruit segments
2 tablespoons sunflower seeds (raw or toasted; see page 112)

Lunch

Pasta and Broccoli Salad (see page 115)

Snack

1 cup plain low-fat yogurt
6 whole almonds (may be stirred into yogurt)

Dinner

Spicy Rice and Beans (see page 119)
2 ears steamed corn (each 6 inches long)
Substitute salt (see page 56), if desired

Snack

1 peach (2 3/4 inches across, about the size of a baseball)

❖   ❖

Day 3, Men
Low-calorie, low-carbohydrate
1200 calories

Breakfast

White Omelet with Mushrooms and Cheese (see page 113)

Snack

1 orange (2 1/2 inches across)

Lunch (combine for a sandwich):

2 thin (1 ounce each) slices turkey

2 slices rye bread

Lettuce, if desired

1 teaspoon mayonnaise

Snack

1 cup cantaloupe cubes

1 tablespoon sunflower seeds (raw or toasted; see page 112)

Dinner

Lemon-Baked Bluefish (see page 121)

*1 cup steamed broccoli, seasoned with Lemon-Parsley Dressing
(see page 105)*

1 cup skim milk

1 small whole-grain muffin

2 teaspoons butter

Snack

1 banana (9 inches)

2 tablespoons sunflower seeds (raw or toasted; see page 112)

❖   ❖

Day 4, Men
High-calorie, high-carbohydrate
1700 calories

Breakfast

1 ¹/₂ cups cooked Oatmeal (see page 111)

2 tablespoons raisins

1 cup skim milk

Snack

1 large carrot

2 stalks celery

2 cubes (2 inches each) Corn Bread (see page 112)

Lunch

1 tablespoon sunflower seeds (raw or toasted; see page 112)

1 cup plain low-fat yogurt

1 whole wheat bagel

Snack

1 cup unsweetened apple juice

8 whole-wheat breadsticks (4 inches long by ¹/₂ inch in diameter)

Dinner

Fettuccine and Green Beans with Garlic Sauce (see page 121)

Snack

1 orange (2 ¹/₂ inches across)

4 whole walnuts

❖   ❖

Day 5, Men
Low-calorie, low-carbohydrate
1200 calories

Breakfast

1 cup skim milk

Toast made with 2 thick (³/4-inch) slices whole-grain "homemade" bread (available in health-food stores)

2 teaspoons sugar-free jam or jelly

Snack

¹/2 cup orange juice (fresh or from concentrate, no sugar added)

Lunch

Salmon Salad (see page 117)

Snack

2 tablespoons raisins

1 tablespoon sunflower seeds (raw or toasted; see page 112)

Dinner

Oven-Basted Fish Fillet (see page 122)

1 small whole-grain roll

2 cups raw vegetables for salad

1 to 2 tablespoons low-calorie salad dressing

Snack

1 peach (2³/4 inches across)

❖   ❖

Day 6, Men
High-calorie, high-carbohydrate
1700 calories

Breakfast

6 *Whole Wheat 'n' Honey Pancakes (see page 113)*

1/2 cup unsweetened applesauce

1 cup skim milk

Snack

1 to 2 cups raw-vegetable mix: celery, radish, cucumber, green pepper, etc.

2 tablespoons sunflower seeds (raw or toasted; see page 112)

Lunch

Corn Pasta with Mixed Vegetables (see page 116)

Snack

1/2 medium grapefruit

Dinner

Two-Bean Toss (see page 122)

Snack

1 cup plain low-fat yogurt

1 small pear

Day 7
Low-calorie, low-carbohydrate
1200 calories

Breakfast

1 cup plain low-fat yogurt

1/3 cup uncooked oat bran

3/4 cup blueberries

Snack

1 cup tomato juice

1 tablespoon sunflower seeds (raw or toasted; see page 112)

Lunch (combine for a sandwich):

2 ounces chicken

2 slices whole-grain bread

Lettuce, if desired

1 teaspoon mayonnaise

1 large raw carrot

Snack

1/2 medium grapefruit

Dinner

Ginger Beef and Vegetable Stir-fry (see page 123)

Snack

1 banana (9 inches)

Day 8, Men
High-calorie, high-carbohydrate
1700 calories

Breakfast

1 cup cooked Kashi (see page 114)

1 cup skim milk

1 medium grapefruit

Snack

3/4 cup raw blueberries (or 1 fruit equivalent)

Lunch

Sesame-Bean Sandwich (see page 118)

Snack

2 tablespoons sunflower seeds (raw or toasted; see page 112)

1 raw green bell pepper, medium

Dinner

Sesame-and-Buckwheat Noodles (see page 123)

2 cups steamed and chopped vegetables of choice: onion, green bell pepper, green beans, snow peas, cauliflower, etc.

1 tablespoon soy sauce

Sesame Salt (see page 56), to taste

Snack

2 plums (each 2 inches across)

Day 9, Men
Low-calorie, low-carbohydrate
1200 calories

Breakfast

¹/₂ whole-wheat bagel

2 teaspoons sugar-free jam or jelly

1 cup skim milk

1 tablespoon raisins

Snack

1 orange (2 ¹/₂ inches across)
1 tablespoon sunflower seeds (raw or toasted; see page 112)

Lunch (combine for a salad):

Salad greens (those listed as free foods)
4 medium sardines canned in sild oil (natural sardine oil)
¹/₄ cup low-fat cottage cheese
Durkee's Red Hot Sauce

Snack

¹/₂ whole-wheat bagel
2 teaspoons sugar-free jam or jelly

Dinner

Steamed Shrimp (see page 124)
1 cup steamed spinach combined with vinegar to taste
2 cups raw vegetables combined with 1 tablespoon salad dressing

Snack

4 medium apricots
1 cup plain low-fat yogurt

Day 10, Men
High-calorie, high-carbohydrate
1700 calories

Breakfast

1 cup Granola (see page 114)

1 cup skim milk

4 rings dried apple

Snack

1 orange (2½ inches across)

Lunch

Herbed Pasta-Vegetable Medley (see page 118)

2 cups cooked pasta

Snack

15 grapes (red or green)

Dinner

New Potatoes with Dilled Vegetables (see page 124)

½ cup tomato juice

Snack

⅛ medium honeydew melon, cubed

1 cup plain low-fat yogurt

1 tablespoon sunflower seeds (raw or toasted; see page 112)

Day 11, Men
Low-calorie, low-carbohydrate
1200 calories

Breakfast

2 small whole-grain rolls

2 teaspoons sugar-free jam or jelly

1 cup skim milk

Snack

1/2 medium grapefruit

Lunch (combine for a sandwich):

3 ounces cooked lean ground beef

1 pita (6 inches across)

Salad greens: celery, cucumber, radish, onion, and mushrooms with lemon juice and herbs, if desired

Snack

4 rings dried apple

Dinner

Chicken-Shallot Sauté (see page 125)

2 cups raw vegetables for salad

2 teaspoons salad dressing

Snack

1 cup plain low-fat yogurt

Day 12, Men
High-calorie, high-carbohydrate
1700 calories

Breakfast

2 Oat-Bran Muffins (see page 115)
1 cup plain low-fat yogurt

Snack

1 orange (2 1/2 inches across)

Lunch

Sweet-Potato Treat (see page 119)
2 slices whole-grain bread
1/4 cup low-fat cottage cheese
1 teaspoon butter

Snack

1 red or green bell pepper, 1 small cucumber, 1/4 avocado
(all chopped and combined with vinegar or lemon juice and
herb seasoning)
3 breadsticks (4 inches long by 1/2 inch in diameter)

Dinner

Five-spice Noodles with Chick-peas (see page 125)

Snack

4 rings dried apple

Day 13, Men
Low-calorie, low-carbohydrate
1200 calories

Breakfast

1 cup ready-to-eat unsweetened cereal
(such as Nutri-Grain Almond Raisin)

1 cup skim milk

1 banana (9 inches)

Snack

1 orange (2 1/2 inches across)

Lunch

1/2 cup canned salmon

Free salad greens

2 teaspoons mayonnaise

Snack

1 large tomato

Lettuce

Dinner

Sautéed Turkey with Asparagus and Pea Pods (see page 126)

2 cups raw vegetables for salad

Lemon-Parsley Dressing (see page 105)

Snack

1 small apple

1 cup plain low-fat yogurt

Day 14, Men
High-calorie, high-carbohydrate
1700 calories

Breakfast

1/2 cup cooked beans of your choice

2 slices whole-grain bread

1 cup tomato juice

Snack

2 tablespoons sunflower seeds (raw or toasted; see page 112)

1 orange (2 1/2 inches across)

Lunch (combine for a sandwich):

1 tablespoon peanut butter

9 cucumber slices

Bean sprouts

2 teaspoons mayonnaise

2 slices cracked-wheat bread or any whole-grain bread

Snack

1 cup assorted raw vegetables

1 cup skim milk

Dinner

Potato Salad (see page 126)

1 cup brown rice

Snack

1 banana (9 inches)

WOMEN'S 1200-CALORIE ALTERNATING
PLAN

The following menus provide three meals and three snacks a day for fourteen days. The reducing plan consists of a diet that averages 1200 calories, alternating between 1000- and 1400-calorie days.

Day 1, Women
Low-calorie, low-carbohydrate
1000 calories

Breakfast

French Toast with Applesauce (see page 111)

Snack

1 cup skim milk

Lunch

Tuna Salad (see page 116)
1 large tomato, sliced

Snack

1 pita (6 inches across)
Salad greens: endive, escarole, spinach, lettuce, romaine

Dinner

2 ounces lean broiled steak (cooked weight)
1 small (3-ounce) baked potato
Dilled Zucchini (see page 120)

Snack

15 grapes (red or green)

❖   ❖

Day 2, Women
High-calorie, high-carbohydrate
1400 calories

Breakfast

²/₃ *cup concentrated uncooked bran cereal (should contain little
or no sugar, such as Kellogg's All Bran with extra fiber)*

1 cup skim milk (use desired amount on cereal and drink the rest)

Snack

¹/₂ medium grapefruit or ³/₄ cup grapefruit segments

2 tablespoons sunflower seeds (raw or toasted; see page 112)

Lunch

Pasta and Broccoli Salad (see page 115)

Snack

1 cup plain low-fat yogurt

6 whole almonds (may be stirred into yogurt)

Dinner

Spicy Rice and Beans (see page 119)

2 ears steamed corn (each 6 inches long)

Substitute salt (see page 56), if desired

Snack

1 peach (2³/₄ inches across, about the size of a baseball)

❖   ❖

Day 3, Women
Low-calorie, low-carbohydrate
1000 calories

Breakfast

White Omelet with Mushrooms and Cheese (see page 113)

Snack

1 orange (2½ inches across)

Lunch (combine for a sandwich):

2 thin (1 ounce each) slices turkey

1 slice rye bread

Lettuce

1 teaspoon mayonnaise

Snack

1 cup cantaloupe cubes

1 tablespoon sunflower seeds (raw or toasted; see page 112)

Dinner

Lemon-Baked Bluefish (see page 121)

*1 cup steamed broccoli, seasoned with Lemon-Parsley Dressing
(see page 105)*

1 cup skim milk

1 small whole-grain muffin

1 teaspoon butter

Snack

1 banana (9 inches)

1 tablespoon sunflower seeds (raw or toasted; see page 112)

Day 4, Women
High-calorie, high-carbohydrate
1400 calories

Breakfast

1 cup cooked Oatmeal (see page 111)

2 tablespoons raisins

1 cup skim milk

Snack

1 large carrot

2 stalks celery

1 cube (2 inches) Corn Bread (see page 112)

Lunch

1 tablespoon sunflower seeds (raw or toasted; see page 112)

1 cup plain low-fat yogurt

1 whole-wheat bagel

Snack

1/2 cup unsweetened apple juice

6 whole-wheat breadsticks (4 inches long by 1/2 inch in diameter)

Dinner

Fettuccine and Green Beans with Garlic Sauce (see page 121)

Snack

1 orange (2 1/2 inches across)

4 whole walnuts

❖   ❖

Day 5, Women
Low-calorie, low-carbohydrate
1000 calories

Breakfast

1 cup skim milk

2 slices whole-grain bread, toasted

2 teaspoons sugar-free jam or jelly

Snack

1/2 cup orange juice (fresh or from concentrate, no sugar added)

Lunch

Salmon Salad (see page 117)

Snack

2 tablespoons raisins

Dinner

Oven-Basted Fish Fillet (see page 122)

1 small whole-grain roll

2 cups raw vegetables for salad

1 to 2 tablespoons low-calorie salad dressing

Snack

1 peach (2 3/4 inches across)

❖   ❖

❖   ❖

Day 6, Women
High-calorie, high-carbohydrate
1400 calories

Breakfast

4 Whole Wheat 'n' Honey Pancakes (see page 113)

1/2 cup unsweetened applesauce

1 cup skim milk

Snack

*1 to 2 cups raw-vegetable mix: celery, radish, cucumber,
green pepper, etc.*

1 tablespoon sunflower seeds (raw or toasted; see page 112)

Lunch

Corn Pasta with Mixed Vegetables (see page 116)

Snack

1/2 medium grapefruit

Dinner

Two-Bean Toss (see page 122)

Snack

1 cup plain low-fat yogurt

1 small pear

❖   ❖

Day 7, Women
Low-calorie, low-carbohydrate
1000 calories

Breakfast

1 cup plain low-fat yogurt

1/3 cup uncooked oat bran

3/4 cup blueberries

Snack

1 cup tomato juice

1 tablespoon sunflower seeds (raw or toasted; see page 112)

Lunch (combine for a sandwich):

2 ounces chicken

1 slice whole-grain bread

Lettuce, if desired

1 teaspoon mayonnaise

1 large raw carrot

Snack

1/2 medium grapefruit

Dinner

Ginger Beef and Vegetable Stir-fry (see page 123)

Snack

1 banana (9 inches)

❖   ❖

Day 8, Women
High-calorie, high-carbohydrate
1400 calories

Breakfast

1 cup cooked Kashi (see page 114)

1 cup skim milk

1 medium grapefruit

Snack

¾ cup raw blueberries (or 1 fruit equivalent)

Lunch

Sesame-Bean Sandwich (see page 118)

Snack

1 tablespoon sunflower seeds (raw or toasted; see page 112)

1 raw green bell pepper, medium

Dinner

Sesame-and-Buckwheat Noodles (see page 123)

*2 cups steamed and chopped vegetables of your choice: onion,
bell pepper, green beans, snow peas, cauliflower, etc., with:*

1 tablespoon soy sauce

Sesame Salt (see page 56), as desired

Snack

2 plums (each 2 inches across)

❖   ❖

Day 9, Women
Low-calorie, low-carbohydrate
1000 calories

Breakfast

1/2 whole-wheat bagel

2 teaspoons sugar-free jam or jelly

1 cup skim milk

1 tablespoon raisins

Snack

1 orange (2 1/2 inches across)

Lunch (combine for a salad):

Salad greens (those listed as free foods)
4 medium sardines canned in sild oil (natural sardine oil)
1/4 cup low-fat cottage cheese
Durkee's Red Hot Sauce

Snack

1/2 whole-wheat bagel
2 teaspoons sugar-free jam or jelly

Dinner

Steamed Shrimp (see page 124)
1 cup steamed spinach, with vinegar to taste
2 cups raw vegetables for salad
1 tablespoon salad dressing

Snack

4 medium apricots

❖   ❖

Day 10, Women
High-calorie, high-carbohydrate
1400 calories

Breakfast

¹/₂ cup Granola (see page 114)

1 cup skim milk

4 rings dried apple

Snack

1 orange (2¹/₂ inches across)

Lunch

Herbed Pasta-Vegetable Medley (see page 118)

Snack

15 grapes (red or green)

Dinner

New Potatoes with Dilled Vegetables (see page 124)

¹/₂ cup tomato juice

Snack

¹/₈ medium honeydew melon, cubed

1 cup plain low-fat yogurt

1 tablespoon sunflower seeds (raw or toasted; see page 112)

❖   ❖

Day 11, Women
Low-calorie, low-carbohydrate
1000 calories

Breakfast

1 small whole-grain roll

2 teaspoons sugar-free jam or jelly

1 cup skim milk

Snack

1/2 medium grapefruit

Lunch (combine for a sandwich):

3 ounces cooked lean ground beef

1 pita (6 inches across)

*Salad greens: celery, cucumber, radish, onion, and mushrooms,
with lemon juice and herbs if desired*

Snack

4 rings dried apple

Dinner

Chicken-Shallot Sauté (see page 125)

2 cups raw vegetables for salad

2 teaspoons salad dressing

Snack

1 cup assorted vegetables

❖   ❖

Day 12, Women
High-calorie, high-carbohydrate
1400 calories

Breakfast

2 small Oat-Bran Muffins (see page 115)

1 cup plain low-fat yogurt

Snack

1 orange (2 1/2 inches across)

Lunch

1 Sweet-Potato Treat (see page 119)

1 slice whole-grain bread

1/4 cup low-fat cottage cheese

Snack (combine for a salad):

1 red or green bell pepper, 1 small cucumber, 1/4 avocado (all chopped and combined with vinegar or lemon juice and herb seasoning)

2 breadsticks (4 inches long by 1/2 inch in diameter)

Dinner

Five-spice Noodles with Chick-peas (see page 125)

Snack

4 rings dried apple

❖   ❖

Day 13, Women
Low-calorie, low-carbohydrate
1000 calories

Breakfast

*3/4 cup ready-to-eat unsweetened cereal
(such as Nutri-Grain Almond Raisin)*

1 cup skim milk

1 banana (9 inches)

Snack

1 orange (2 1/2 inches across)

Lunch

1/2 cup canned salmon

Free salad greens

1 teaspoon mayonnaise

Snack

1 large tomato

Lettuce

Dinner

Sautéed Turkey with Asparagus and Pea Pods (see page 126)

2 cups raw vegetables for salad

Lemon-Parsley Dressing (see page 105)

Snack

1 small apple

❖   ❖

Day 14, Women
High-calorie, high-carbohydrate
1400 calories

Breakfast

1/2 cup cooked beans of your choice

2 slices whole-grain bread

1 cup tomato juice

Snack

1 tablespoon sunflower seeds (raw or toasted; see page 112)

1 orange (2 1/2 inches across)

Lunch (combine for a sandwich):

1 tablespoon peanut butter

9 cucumber slices

Bean sprouts

1 teaspoon mayonnaise

2 slices cracked-wheat bread or any whole-grain bread

Snack

1 cup assorted raw vegetables

1 cup skim milk

Dinner

Potato Salad (see page 126)

Snack

1 banana (9 inches)

❖   ❖

DAILY SUPPLEMENTS

The Recommended Dietary Allowances (RDAs) represent the optimal "dosages" of certain micronutrients that most people need for good health; as we explained in the first part of this book, any calorie-restricted diet is likely to be deficient in some of these nutrients.

Nevertheless, the Princeton Plan is much more complete in these and other nutrients than the average American diet. In fact, averaged over the two-day alternating plan, the Plan meets or comes close to meeting the needs for vitamins A, C, and E, as well as for calcium and magnesium. It *may* be somewhat low, however, for sodium, potassium, zinc, and some other trace elements and vitamins. (We say "may" be low because the RDAs are set purposely high: An amount below the RDA does not necessarily represent a deficiency.)

Averaged over the fourteen days of the Plan, the diet is very well balanced, and anyone who follows it for an extended period of time will become and remain very healthy. Nevertheless, to make certain that all your nutritional needs are met, we recommend certain daily supplements. To obtain all of our recommended nutrients, it's likely that you would need to take three different supplements: a multivitamin-B complex, an antioxidant, and a multimineral formula. When choosing your own supplements, look for ones that, when combined, contain all the micronutrients we list, in as close as possible to the recommended dosages. To make it easier to obtain all the listed micronutrients, we have developed two special formulas: The Princeton Plan A.M. Formula (which contains all the nutrients listed under "Multivitamin-B Complex" and "Antioxidant Formula," page 100) and The Princeton Plan P.M. Formula (which contains all the nutrients listed under "Multimineral Formula," page 101). These two formulas are available in many pharmacies and health stores. To help you locate a store in your area that carries them, call (800) 635-4631. Note that The Princeton Plan A.M. and P.M. Formulas are different from the Princeton Plan HC and LC Powdered Diet Drinks mentioned on page 32.

The vitamins and minerals in these three supplements will work together with the nutrients in your food to ensure that your body has all the raw materials it needs to make "good" prostaglandins and to produce thermogenesis for continuing weight loss. In addition, the antioxidants will help protect all your body's cells from free-radical damage, which increases with exercise. For information on additional supplements to further increase thermogenesis, see chapter 19.

Please take the supplements at the times indicated, because some vitamins and minerals can interfere with one another's absorption when taken simultaneously.

MULTIVITAMIN-B COMPLEX (TO BE TAKEN WITH BREAKFAST)

B_1	10 mg.
B_2	10 mg.
B_3	20 mg.
B_6	10 mg.
B_{12}	50 mg.
Folic acid	400 mcg.
Pantothenic acid	10 mg.

ANTIOXIDANT FORMULA (TO BE TAKEN WITH BREAKFAST)

Selenium	100 mcg.
Vitamin C	250 mg.
Vitamin E	200 IU
Vitamin A	4,000 to 5,000 IU
Vitamin D	200 IU
Beta-carotene	10,000 IU

MULTIMINERAL FORMULA (TO BE TAKEN WITH DINNER)

Magnesium	100 mg.
Calcium	200 mg.
Iron	10 mg.
Copper	*no more than* 1 mg.
Zinc	15 mg.
Manganese	5 mg.
Chromium	200 mcg.

FREE FOODS

A free food is any food or drink that contains fewer than 20 calories per serving. Between or during meals you may enjoy as much as you like of those items that have no serving size specified. You may have two or three servings per day of starred items in the serving size specified.

Drinks
Bouillon or broth without fat
Bouillon, low-sodium
Carbonated drinks, sugar-free
Carbonated water
Club soda
Cocoa powder, unsweetened (1 tablespoon)*
Coffee/Tea (see page 40 for possible warnings about caffeine)
Tonic water, sugar-free

Nonstick Pan Spray

Fruit
Cranberries, unsweetened (½ cup)*
Rhubarb, unsweetened (½ cup)

Vegetables (raw or steamed, 1 cup)*
Cabbage, red or green
Celery
Chinese cabbage
Cucumber
Daikon
Green onion
Hot peppers
Mushrooms
Radishes
Sprouts
Zucchini

Salad Greens
Arugula

Endive
Escarole
Lettuce, all kinds (iceberg, ro-
    maine, Boston, Bibb, etc.)
Radicchio
Spinach

Sweet Substitutes
Gelatin, sugar-free
Gum, sugar-free
Jam or Jelly, sugar-free (2 tea-
    spoons)*
Sugar substitutes (saccharin, as-
    partame)

Condiments
Catsup (1 tablespoon)*

Horseradish
Mustard
Pickles, dill, unsweetened
Salad dressing, no-calorie type
    (2 tablespoons)*
Taco sauce (1 tablespoon)*
Vinegar

Seasonings
All herbs
Flavoring extracts
Garlic and garlic powder
Hot-pepper sauce (capsicum)
Lemon and lime juice
Soy sauce (1 tablespoon)*
Wine, in cooking (1/4 cup)*
Worcestershire sauce

BEVERAGES

The following beverages may all be enjoyed on the Princeton Eating
Plan. If you drink milk or fruit juice, you must include the drink within
the allowed daily food exchanges. For information on using the exchange lists, see chapter 10, "Your Personal Eating Plan."

Cold Beverages
Bottled water
Milk, skim, 1- or 2-percent fat
Mineral water
Pure tap water
Seltzer water
Sugar-free fruit juices
Water with splash of lemon or
    fruit juice

Hot Beverages
Grain coffee substitutes
Herbal teas
Hot apple juice
Hot water with lemon or lime
    juice
Postum
Real coffee or tea

THE PRINCETON PLAN
RECIPES

THE recipes that follow are for dishes indicated in capital letters in the two-week menu plan.

Some recipes, such as those for broiled fish and meats, are simply healthful ways of preparing standard American fare. Others, including some bean and pasta dishes, may be more unfamiliar. You may at first find it strange to eat so much carbohydrate at one meal, but remember that these menus were planned to promote maximum stimulation of thermogenesis for speedy weight loss. Since every calorie contributes to optimal nutrition as well as to metabolic stimulation, it's important to eat all foods listed for each day's meals.

All of the lunch recipes are designed to be "portable"—that is, you can prepare them the night before and take them to work the next day in a container. All pasta dishes, unless noted otherwise, are equally good hot or cold.

Remember that you are free to change suggested seasonings in any recipe or to add your own favorite spices and herbs. We especially recommend hot-red-pepper products for their thermogenic effect; they enhance a number of dishes that may not include them in the list of ingredients. Bear in mind also that free foods (see pages 101–102) may be added to any dish.

Although not all recipes call for the use of PAM, it may be used any time to prevent sticking. You may also add Butter Buds to any dish, *in moderation.*

Except where noted, recipes are for a single serving; double the amounts for two.

Cooked Pasta

Twists, shells, and other pasta shapes yield close to the same amount cooked as when dry. Simply cook ¼ cup less dry pasta than the cooked amount called for in the recipe.

It is more difficult to estimate cooked amounts of pasta when dealing with strands (spaghetti, fettuccine, etc.). A bundle about the diameter of a broomstick yields one cup cooked. The first few times you cook a given amount, you may want to measure the cooked pasta. Leftover cold pasta tastes great in salads and may be reheated in the microwave oven with no loss in texture.

Cooking times depend upon the thickness of the pasta and the type of flour from which it was made. Pastas may require anywhere from 8 to 15 minutes to cook thoroughly. Be sure to read the directions on the package.

To cook: Fill a 2-quart saucepan ⅔ to ¾ full of water. Bring water to a rolling boil. Add the pasta, vigorously stirring to separate (cooking chopsticks are a good stirring tool). Return to a boil. Boil, uncovered, stirring periodically, for 8 to 10 minutes or until desired tenderness is reached. Do not overcook. Drain and rinse under hot running water. Serve immediately.

DRESSINGS AND SAUCES

Sesame Dressing

½ cup oil of your choice
¼ cup toasted sesame seeds
2 tablespoons lemon juice
2 tablespoons vinegar

½ teaspoon salt
1 cup chopped fresh parsley
(optional)

Put all ingredients in blender and blend until nearly smooth. Refrigerate. This dressing is especially good with steamed veggies and/or pasta.

Yield: 1/2 to 3/4 cup

Lemon-Parsley Dressing

1/2 cup oil of your choice
2 teaspoons cider vinegar
3 tablespoons freshly squeezed
*   lemon juice*
1 cup fresh parsley

1/4 teaspoon dried marjoram
2 teaspoons chopped green bell
*   pepper*
Dash pepper

Place all ingredients in blender and blend until parsley is chopped fine. This dressing is good with veggies, meats, fish, and pasta.

Yield: about 1 cup

Curry Dressing

1 cup oil of your choice
1/2 cup wine vinegar
1/2 teaspoon salt (optional)

1/4 teaspoon mustard powder
1/4 teaspoon curry powder

Shake all ingredients together in a covered jar. This dressing is great with potatoes or as an unusual salad dressing.

Yield: 1 1/2 cups

French Dressing

1/2 cup oil of your choice
2 tablespoons lemon juice
2 tablespoons cider or wine
  vinegar

1/4 teaspoon paprika
1/4 teaspoon salt
1/4 teaspoon mustard powder
Dash cayenne pepper

Shake all ingredients together in a covered jar. This is a classic salad dressing.

Yield: 3/4 cup

Greek Dressing

1/3 cup safflower oil
1/3 cup olive oil
2 tablespoons lemon juice
2 tablespoons wine vinegar
2 cloves garlic
2 tablespoons plain low-fat
  yogurt

1 tablespoon prepared mustard
1/2 teaspoon salt
1/4 teaspoon dried sage
1/4 teaspoon dried thyme
1/4 teaspoon dried basil
1/4 teaspoon dried oregano

Combine all ingredients in blender and blend. Store in a covered jar in the refrigerator. This dressing is delicious on salads and with pasta.

Yield: approximately 1 cup

Creamy Dressing

Instead of mayonnaise or sour cream, add 1 to 2 tablespoons of low-fat yogurt, buttermilk, tofu, or cottage cheese to any dressing recipe. In a blender or food processor, mix the dressing briefly for a smooth texture.

Salsa

3 ripe tomatoes
3 tablespoons olive oil
1 medium onion
1 large carrot
1 small green chili, minced
2 jalapeño peppers, minced
1 small red bell pepper, minced
1 stalk celery

2 tablespoons apple-cider
vinegar
3 tablespoons fresh cilantro
(coriander leaf), minced
1 clove garlic, minced
1 teaspoon dried oregano
1 teaspoon powdered cumin
1/2 teaspoon black pepper

Remove skins from tomatoes by plunging them in boiling water for a few seconds, then peeling. Chop tomatoes into small cubes and set aside in a bowl. Heat oil in large skillet. Add onion and sauté until it begins to soften. Add carrot, chili, jalapeño peppers, red pepper, celery, and vinegar, and sauté for 5 minutes, stirring frequently. Stir in cilantro, garlic, oregano, cumin, and black pepper. Sauté mixture 2 minutes more. Allow vegetables to cool slightly; then add to tomatoes and mix well.

Salsa can be used to add zip to soups, meat, pasta, omelets, or even on salads for a "taco" flavor.

Yield: 4 cups

Tomato Sauce

1 diced onion
1 clove garlic, minced
1 stalk celery, diced
1 green bell pepper, diced
1 carrot, diced
1/4 cup oil of choice
2 cups chopped tomatoes (fresh
or canned), drained

1 teaspoon salt
1 teaspoon dried oregano
1/2 teaspoon crushed black
peppercorns
1 bay leaf
2 tablespoons chopped fresh
parsley (optional)

In a 2-quart saucepan, sauté onion, garlic, celery, green pepper, and carrot in oil for 5 to 10 minutes. Add remaining ingredients and mix well. Cover pot and cook over medium-low heat for 10 minutes, stirring occasionally. Before serving, remove the bay leaf and add chopped parsley, if desired.

This basic tomato-sauce recipe may be served with pasta, rice, lamb, beef, pork, fish, broiled eggplant, or omelets.

Yield: approximately 4 cups

GRAINS AND BEANS

Beans, Peas, and Lentils

Beans are one food in which the nutritional value of the canned product is equivalent to the nutritional value of the home-prepared product; and, since they are precooked, canned beans can be added immediately to whatever you are preparing. When using canned beans, remember to rinse them in a colander to remove excess sodium.

There are four methods for cooking beans from scratch. For all of them, first place the dried beans in a colander and rinse them well. Split peas and lentils may then be cooked directly; other beans must first be soaked or otherwise prepared, as follows:

1. *Presoak method.* Presoaking cuts down cooking time by about
   ½ hour. However, because some vitamins and minerals will
   pass into the water, be sure to cook the beans in the soaking
   water. To soak, place beans in a bowl and cover them with
   water, allowing about 2 to 3 inches of extra water (the beans
   will expand). Soybeans should be refrigerated during presoaking to prevent fermentation. Soak for approximately 1 hour.
   When the beans have finished soaking, pour them, with the
   water, into a saucepan or Dutch oven. Add more water if
   necessary to cover the beans. Bring them to a boil, then lower
   the heat and simmer with the lid slightly ajar over the pot to
   prevent boiling over. Check the beans from time to time and

add more water if needed. Remember that the beans must be kept covered with liquid at all times.

2. *Quickboil method.* Presoaking is unnecessary if the rinsed, dried legumes are quickly washed and dropped into boiling water so slowly that the boiling does not stop. When all the beans have been added, quickly lower the heat so that the protein in the beans does not become tough. Cook as in method 1.

3. *Overnight method.* Soak the beans overnight, then bring them slowly to a boil in the water used for soaking. Reduce heat and simmer as in method 1.

4. *Crockpot method.* Place the rinsed beans in the crockpot, fill it with water to within 2 or 3 inches of the top of the pot, then cook on high for 4 to 6 hours or overnight, depending on the type of bean.

Yield per cup of dried bean will vary depending on the type of bean. Generally 1 cup of dried beans will yield 2 cups cooked. See the chart on page 110 for more information.

The cooking time for dried beans, peas, and lentils varies widely. It may be anywhere from 45 minutes for lentils to 2½ hours or more for soybeans (see chart on page 110 for approximate cooking times of most beans). If the beans are being prepared for a salad or for a dish where they should remain intact, cook them until just tender. For soups, pasta dishes, or when mixed with steamed vegetables, beans should be cooked more thoroughly. That is, when a cooked bean is placed on your tongue and pushed against the roof of your mouth, it should mash easily.

Brown Rice

Natural brown rice is tasty and more nutritious than white rice. When possible, purchase rice (or any other grain) that is organically grown. Supermarkets carry brown rice, though it's not necessarily organically grown.

To cook: Rinse 1 cup of brown rice in cold water and drain well.

COOKING TIMES AND PROPORTION FOR GRAINS AND BEANS

Grain (1 Cup Dry Measure)	Water	Cooking Time	Yield
Barley (whole)	3 cups	1 hour 15 minutes	3½ cups
Brown rice	2 cups	1 hour	3 cups
Buckwheat (kasha)	2 cups	15 minutes	2½ cups
Bulgur wheat	2 cups	15–20 minutes	2½ cups
Cracked wheat	2 cups	25 minutes	2⅓ cups
Millet	3 cups	45 minutes	3½ cups
Coarse cornmeal (polenta)	4 cups	25 minutes	3 cups
Wild rice	3 cups	1 hour or more	4 cups
Whole wheat berries	3 cups	2 hours	2⅔ cups
Quinoa	2 cups	15 minutes	2½ cups
Black beans	4 cups	1½ hours	2 cups
Black-eyed peas	3 cups	1 hour	2 cups
Garbanzos (chick-peas)	4 cups	3 hours	2 cups
Great northern beans	3½ cups	2 hours	2 cups
Kidney beans	3 cups	1½ hours	2 cups
Lentils and split peas	3 cups	45 minutes	2¼ cups
Limas	2 cups	1½ hours	1¼ cups
Baby limas	2 cups	1½ hours	1¾ cups
Pinto beans	3 cups	2½ hours	2 cups
Red beans	3 cups	3 hours	2 cups
Small white beans (navy, etc.)	3 cups	2½ hours	2 cups
Soybeans	4 cups	3 hours or more	2 cups
Soy grits	2 cups	15 minutes	2 cups

From *The New Laurel's Kitchen* by Laurel Robertson, Carol Flinders, and Brian Ruppenthal, © 1976, 1986 by The Blue Mountain Center of Meditation. Published by Ten Speed Press, Berkeley, Calif.

Bring 2 cups of water to a boil. Slowly pour in the rice, stirring as you pour. When the water returns to a boil, turn the heat down as low as possible. Cover and cook slowly until all the water is absorbed, approximately 45 minutes to 1 hour.

Yield: 3 cups

For other grains, prepare as for brown rice. See the chart on page 110 for amounts and cooking times.

BREAKFAST AND SNACK RECIPES

French Toast with Applesauce

¼ cup skim milk   *Ground cinnamon*
1 medium egg, slightly beaten   *½ cup unsweetened applesauce*
1 or 2 slices whole-grain bread

Spray a nonstick pan with PAM. Heat to medium. While waiting for the pan to heat, combine skim milk with egg. Dip bread into milk-egg mixture. Place soaked bread in pan along with any extra milk-egg mixture. Cook on both sides until golden brown. Serve hot. Sprinkle with cinnamon. Applesauce may be used as a topping if desired.

Yield: 1 serving

Oatmeal

Men	*Women*
¾ cup old-fashioned oats	*½ cup old-fashioned oats*
¼ teaspoon salt	*⅛ teaspoon salt*
1½ cups water	*1 cup water*

Stir oats into briskly boiling water to which salt has already been added. Cook for 5 minutes, stirring occasionally. Cover and remove from heat. Let stand until oatmeal is the consistency you like.

Oats may also be microwaved. Combine water, salt, and old-fashioned oats in a cereal bowl. Microwave at medium power for 5 to 6 minutes or until thickened. Mix before serving. (*Taste tip:* For more flavor, sprinkle cinnamon or Butter Buds on cooked cereal.)

Yield (for men): 1 1/2 cups   *Yield (for women): 1 cup*

Corn Bread

2 cups cornmeal	1 tablespoon brown sugar
1/4 cup wheat germ	1 large egg, beaten
1 teaspoon salt	1 tablespoon oil
1/2 teaspoon baking soda	2 cups low-fat buttermilk
1 teaspoon baking powder	

Preheat oven to 425°F. Oil an 8-inch-square baking pan.

In a large bowl, stir together the dry ingredients. In another bowl, mix the wet ingredients. Combine the two just until they are well mixed. Turn into pan and bake for 20 to 25 minutes. Remove pan to wire rack.

Cut into 2-inch cubes and serve warm, or cool and store, wrapped tightly, in refrigerator.

Toasted Seeds

The flavors of sesame, sunflower, and pumpkin seeds are enhanced by light toasting. There are two slightly different methods that can be used.

Spread seeds in a small, ovenproof casserole dish and place in a 300°F oven for about 20 minutes. Stir often. The less surface area exposed to the heat, the better.

Or, place seeds on an unoiled cookie sheet and put in a 350°F oven for 15 to 20 minutes. No stirring is necessary. This method is easier if you're too busy for frequent stirring.

Remove seeds from oven and let cool. Store in a tightly covered jar in the refrigerator. To prevent rancidity, toast only an amount of seeds that will be used in 2 weeks' time.

White Omelet with Mushrooms and Cheese

3 egg whites

1/4 cup low-fat cottage cheese

1/4 green bell pepper, diced

1/4 small onion, diced

3 mushroom caps, sliced thin

Stir egg whites with a fork. Add cottage cheese and blend together with a fork. Spray a nonstick frying pan with PAM and heat to medium high. Add vegetables and sauté for 2 minutes. Add egg–cottage cheese mixture to sautéed vegetables. Cook until completely set, stirring occasionally with spatula.

Yield: 1 serving

Whole Wheat 'n' Honey Pancakes

1 cup whole-wheat flour

1 teaspoon baking powder

1/2 teaspoon salt

1 egg

1 1/2 cups 2-percent milk

1 1/2 teaspoons honey

1 tablespoon oil

In a medium-size bowl, stir together flour, baking powder, and salt with a fork. In a separate bowl, beat egg slightly and combine with milk and honey. Add this to the dry ingredients and stir briefly. Stir in oil with a few strokes. Use a nonstick griddle or spray griddle with PAM. Heat the griddle until water drops dance when sprinkled on the surface. Slowly spoon batter onto the griddle to make a 4-inch pancake. Cook over medium heat. Turn once when bubbles appear and pop on the surface.

Yield: one dozen 4-inch pancakes

Kashi (Breakfast Pilaf)

Using one packet of Kashi (1 cup uncooked): Bring 2 cups of water to a rolling boil in a 2-quart saucepan. Pour Kashi into the boiling water. Cover for a soft texture or leave uncovered for a slightly chewier texture. Turn heat down until mixture reaches a slow boil (not a simmer). Cook until all the liquid has been absorbed, about 25 minutes. If Kashi is not done, add ¼ cup more liquid and cook until absorbed. Serve hot, with low-fat or skim milk. Unused Kashi may be refrigerated or frozen for future use.

Yield: 3 cups

Granola

Once the theory of making granola is understood, the procedure becomes quite simple. Raw cereal grains are first moistened so that they won't burn, then coated with oil to keep them soft while cooking. The grains are then toasted until they are dry; the oil makes them crunchy. Most people use rolled oats as the base, but other grains can be used.

¼ cup honey	*½ cup raw sunflower seeds*
1 cup water	*¼ cup raw pumpkin seeds*
3 tablespoons vegetable oil	*1 cup bran*
2 teaspoons vanilla extract	*½ cup raw wheat germ*
5 cups rolled oats	*1 teaspoon ground cinnamon*
½ cup broken walnuts	*1 cup raisins*

Preheat oven to 250°F. Combine all ingredients except raisins in a large bowl and stir until well moistened. Spread mixture over the bottom of a large shallow roasting pan or cookie sheet and bake about 1 hour. Stir often with a spatula during baking. Test for doneness by tasting. Baking time will depend upon how thinly the mixture is spread in the pan. Raisins may be added *after* baking.

Yield: about 2½ pounds

Oat-Bran Muffins

2 1/4 cups oat bran

1/4 cup chopped nuts

1/4 cup raisins

1 tablespoon baking powder

1 cup skim milk

1/4 cup honey

2 eggs, beaten

2 tablespoons oil

Preheat oven to 425°F. Line muffin tins with paper baking cups. Combine oat bran, nuts, raisins, and baking powder in a large bowl. In a separate bowl, blend milk, honey, eggs, and oil. Mix wet ingredients with the oat-bran mixture just until dry ingredients are moistened. Fill muffin cups until almost full. Bake for 15 to 17 minutes. Leftover muffins may be frozen.

Yield: 12 muffins

LUNCH RECIPES

Pasta and Broccoli Salad

3/4 cup (for women) or 1 1/4 cups (for men) pasta, dry (twists, shells, or other shapes)

1 stalk broccoli, sliced diagonally into bite-sized pieces (1 cup per serving)

3 tablespoons olive oil

1 tablespoon vinegar

1/2 teaspoon dried oregano

1/2 teaspoon dried basil

1/2 teaspoon salt substitute

1 clove garlic, minced

Pepper to taste

Fill a 2-quart saucepan about 2/3 full with water. Bring to a rolling boil. Stir in pasta. Once water returns to a boil, continue boiling for 7 to 10 minutes or until pasta reaches desired tenderness. Drain and rinse thoroughly with hot, running water.

While pasta is cooking, place broccoli in a vegetable steamer and cover. Steam over boiling water for 5 to 7 minutes or until just tender when pierced with a fork. Remove broccoli from heat and reserve.

While broccoli steams, combine oil, vinegar, oregano, basil, salt substitute, garlic, and pepper in a small jar; cover tightly and shake well.

Combine pasta, broccoli, and dressing (women use 1 tablespoon; men use 2 tablespoons) in a bowl. Toss gently and serve. *Note:* This dish can be prepared the night before and eaten cold.

Yield: 2 cups (1 serving) for women, or 2 1/2 cups (1 serving) for men.

Tuna Salad

1/2 cup white albacore tuna,
*   packed in water*
2 teaspoons safflower-oil
*   mayonnaise (available in*
*   most health-food stores)*

1/4 teaspoon garlic powder
1/4 teaspoon onion powder
1/4 stalk celery, chopped
Juice of half a lemon
Lettuce leaves

Place all ingredients (except lettuce) in a bowl and mix well. Serve on lettuce leaves.

Yield: 1 serving

Corn Pasta with Mixed Vegetables

1/2 cup Tomato Sauce (see page
*   107)*
1 cup cooked wheat-free corn
*   pasta (such as DeBoles Thin*
*   Spaghetti)*

1 1/2 cups steamed and diced
*   mixed vegetables: peas,*
*   carrots, asparagus,*
*   cauliflower, peppers, etc.*
1 teaspoon butter

Make Tomato Sauce according to the recipe. Allow sauce to simmer while preparing pasta and vegetables according to following instructions. (If using a commercial, sugar-free sauce, heat in a saucepan while pasta boils.)

Fill a 2-quart saucepan about ⅔ full of water. Bring to a rolling boil. Stir in corn spaghetti to separate. Return to a boil. Boil uncovered, stirring occasionally, for 9 to 10 minutes or until pasta reaches desired tenderness. Do not overcook. Drain and rinse thoroughly with hot running water.

Choose any nonstarchy vegetables, wash them under cold running water, and slice into bite-size pieces. The amount of all vegetables before steaming should be 2 to 2½ cups. Steam vegetables in a vegetable steamer according to directions on page 51, adding the longer-cooking vegetables first.

Mix tomato sauce and pasta together. The vegetables may be served separately, topped with 1 teaspoon of butter or, if desired, mixed with the pasta and sauce.

Yield: 2½ cups

Salmon Salad

½ cup canned red or pink
    salmon, with bones
1 teaspoon safflower- or
    canola-oil mayonnaise
    (available in most
    health-food stores)
1 small stalk celery, thinly
    sliced on the digonal

1 medium radish, thinly sliced
1 tablespoon lemon juice
¼ teaspoon paprika
¼ teaspoon garlic powder
¼ teaspoon dried thyme
Lettuce leaves
5 cucumber slices (¼-inch
    thick)

Place all ingredients, except lettuce and cucumber slices, in a bowl and mix well. Serve salmon mixture on lettuce leaves and arrange cucumber slices on the side.

Yield: 1 serving

Sesame-Bean Sandwich

2/3 cup cooked kidney beans

1 tablespoon (for women) or 2
  tablespoons (for men) Sesame
  Dressing (see page 104)

2 slices whole-grain bread
  (thick sliced for men)

2 tablespoons grated Parmesan
  cheese

Finely shredded lettuce

Place kidney beans in a bowl and add Sesame Dressing. Mash beans and dressing together with a fork or potato masher. Spread mixture over the top of a piece of whole-grain bread. Sprinkle with grated Parmesan cheese and add the desired amount of shredded lettuce. Cover with the second slice of bread, cut on the diagonal, and enjoy.

Yield: 1 sandwich

Herbed Pasta-Vegetable Medley

1 cup (for women) or 2 cups
  (for men) cooked pasta

1 stalk broccoli, sliced into
  bite-sized pieces

6 medium-size whole
  mushrooms, sliced 1/4-inch
  thick

1 small zucchini, sliced
  horizontally into 1/4-inch
  pieces

1/3 cup canned kidney beans,
  rinsed and drained

Herbal shake of your choice

Prepare pasta according to guidelines on page 104. While pasta boils, clean and slice vegetables. Place broccoli in steamer and steam for 5 minutes over boiling water. Add mushrooms and zucchini and steam 5 minutes more.

Heat kidney beans by adding to boiling pasta 1 minute before end of cooking time. Drain pasta and beans.

Combine pasta, beans, and vegetables. Toss gently. Add the herbal shake of your choice.

Yield: 3 cups for women, or 4 cups for men

Sweet-Potato Treat

1 medium sweet potato   *1 teaspoon butter (optional)*

Scrub sweet potato and cut off woody portions, but leave skin on. Pierce potato with a fork. Bake in a moderate oven (375–400°F) for 50 to 60 minutes, or until done. For a softer texture, wrap sweet potato in aluminum foil before baking. To serve, cut potato in half lengthwise and make a crisscross pattern in the flesh with a fork. Add 1 teaspoon of butter to season, if desired.

Be aware that undercooked sweet potatoes do not taste good; test for doneness by piercing with a fork before removing from oven. Cooking time will vary depending on the size of the sweet potato. Sweet potatoes may be microwaved. Follow your manufacturer's directions.

Yield: 1 serving

DINNER RECIPES

Spicy Rice and Beans

½ cup (for women) or ⅔ cup (for men) cooked kidney beans, rinsed and drained if canned

1 cup cooked brown rice
3 tablespoons Salsa (see page 107)

Cook brown rice according to instructions on page 109. While rice is cooking, prepare Salsa. Five minutes before rice is done, heat beans with salsa. Combine with rice and serve.

Yield: 1 ½ cups for women, or 1 ⅔ cups for men

Oven-Broiled Steak

Select a porterhouse, T-bone, club, sirloin, or tenderloin steak cut 1 to 1½ inches thick. Cut away any visible fat from the edges of the steak. Slash the membrane around the steak at intervals— don't cut into the meat. Place steak on rack of broiler pan. For thin steaks, place near the heat; for thicker steaks, place them farther away. Broil top side. Season with herbal seasoning and pepper. Turn and broil other side until meat is brown and done to your liking.

For 1-inch steak, allow 10 to 15 minutes for rare; 12 to 20 minutes for medium. For 1½-inch steak, allow 15 to 20 minutes for rare; 20 to 30 minutes for medium.

Pan-Broiled Steak

Select a porterhouse, T-bone, club, sirloin, or tenderloin steak. Cut ½- to ¾-inch thick. Place in preheated heavy skillet over medium heat. Do not add fat. Brown on both sides. Season with herbal seasoning and pepper. Finish cooking (do not cover), pouring off fat as it accumulates and turning occasionally. Total cooking time for rare steak is about 6 to 8 minutes; for medium- or well-done steak, 10 to 12 minutes. If desired, season again, and serve.

Dilled Zucchini

1 medium zucchini	1 tablespoon soy sauce
1 tablespoon safflower or sesame oil	1 teaspoon fresh dill

Wash zucchini and remove ends. Slice zucchini into ½-inch cubes. Sauté in oil for 5 minutes over medium heat. Add soy sauce and dill. Cover and simmer over low heat for 5 more minutes.

Yield: 1 serving

Fettucine and Green Beans with Garlic Sauce

1 cup (about 30 strands)   2 teaspoons olive oil
  fettucini, cooked   1/4 teaspoon curry powder
1 cup green beans   1/4 teaspoon garlic powder

Fill a 2-quart saucepan about 2/3 full with water. Bring to a rolling boil. Stir in fettuccine to separate. Return to boil. Boil uncovered, stirring occasionally, for 12 to 15 minutes or until pasta reaches desired tenderness. Do not overcook. Drain and rinse thoroughly with hot running water.

While fettuccine is boiling, prepare beans by removing both ends; then cut in 1-inch-long slices on the diagonal. Steam in vegetable steamer for approximately 5 minutes, or until desired tenderness is reached. Mix olive oil, curry powder, and garlic powder together in a small dish.

Combine fettuccine, beans, and olive-oil dressing. Toss gently and serve.

Yield: 2 cups

Lemon-Baked Bluefish

1 bluefish fillet (3 or 4 ounces   Lemon juice
  raw = 2 or 3 ounces   Pepper to taste
  cooked; see Note)   Lemon and parsley, for garnish

Place bluefish in an oiled baking dish or pan. Sprinkle with lemon juice and pepper and bake at 425°F. Serve with lemon and parsley.

Baking time: Measure the fish at its thickest point. Allow 10 minutes cooking time per inch of thickness. Double the cooking time if the fish is frozen. Fish must be baked in a very hot oven (425 to 450°F).

Note: If bluefish is not available, substitute another fatty fish, such as salmon, mackerel, tuna, sable, or brook trout.

Yield: 1 serving

Two-Bean Toss

*¹⁄₄ cup lima beans, rinsed and
drained if canned*
*¹⁄₃ cup (for women) or ²⁄₃ cup
(for men) red beans*
1 cup cooked brown rice
1 cup steamed broccoli

¹⁄₄ cup oil
¹⁄₄ cup wine vinegar
*¹⁄₈ teaspoon each dried dill,
cumin, red pepper, and basil*
1 tablespoon tomato sauce

Use rinsed and drained canned beans or prepare lima beans and red beans earlier in the day according to instructions on page 108.

Prepare brown rice according to instructions on page 109.

Slice broccoli and steam in a vegetable steamer until tender, about 10 to 12 minutes.

Combine oil, vinegar, herbs, and tomato sauce in a jar. Cover and shake well.

Toss beans, rice, broccoli, and 2 tablespoons dressing together and serve. Remaining dressing may be stored in refrigerator.

Yield: 2¹⁄₂ cups for women, or 3 cups for men

Oven-Basted Fish Fillet

*1 raw fish fillet (5 ounce for
women, or 6 ounce for men)*

*Basting sauce: mustard,
paprika, and parsley*

Preheat the oven to 450°F. Place fish fillet on the oiled rack of a broiling pan. Brush with mustard; add paprika and parsley. Place the broiling pan in the oven so that fish is approximately 2 to 3 inches from the heating unit. If fish is frozen, it will have to be placed lower in the oven to prevent overcooking the surface before the interior is cooked. Leave the oven door ajar unless manufacturer's directions state otherwise. Fish may be basted once or twice during the cooking process. Do not turn fish. Allow 10 minutes cooking time per inch of thickness.

Yield: 1 serving

Sesame-and-Buckwheat Noodles

1 cup (for women) or 2 cups
(for men) cooked buckwheat
noodles

2 teaspoons sesame-seed oil

Preparation is the same as for other pastas, except that cooking time will depend upon the thickness of the noodles. Buckwheat noodles, called *soba,* can be found in most health-food stores. The thinner varieties require only 5 to 8 minutes simmering time. After you have drained the noodles, stir in sesame-seed oil for a very delicate flavor.

Yield: 1 serving

Ginger Beef and Vegetable Stir-fry

1 fillet (3-ounce for women, or
  5 ounce for men) steak
1 tablespoon soy sauce
2 cups raw vegetables: 1 small
  green bell pepper, 1 small
  red bell pepper, 1 fresh red

chile, 1 stick celery, 1 small
  carrot
2 tablespoons oil
2 slices fresh gingerroot
  (shredded)

Slice beef very thinly, cutting across the grain, then cut into narrow strips. (This is easier if the meat is partially frozen.) Place in a dish and add soy sauce. Mix well and let sit at room temperature for about 20 minutes.

Cut peppers, chile, celery, and carrot into narrow strips. Heat a wok or sauté pan and add the oil. Stir-fry beef on high heat until lightly and evenly browned. Remove beef from pan and keep warm. Add vegetables and ginger to pan and stir-fry until soft (about 4 minutes). Return beef to pan and continue to cook on high heat about 1 minute more.

Yield: 1 serving

New Potatoes with Dilled Vegetables

2 or 3 small new potatoes
2 cups raw vegetables: 1
   medium carrot, 1 small
   zucchini, 1 stick celery, 1
   small onion

½ cup fresh or frozen green
   peas
1 teaspoon dried dill
1 tablespoon dressing of your
   choice

Thoroughly scrub potatoes and prick with a fork. Place in a steamer basket over boiling water; cover pot, and steam for 10 minutes. In the meantime, peel vegetables and cut into julienne (matchstick) strips. Arrange over potatoes, add peas, and sprinkle dill on top. Cover the pot and steam for 10 more minutes or until potatoes and vegetables are tender. Remove from the pot and spoon dressing over vegetables.

Yield: 1 serving

Steamed Shrimp

6 ounces shrimp

1 teaspoon butter, optional

Wash shrimp thoroughly but do not remove the shells.

Place shrimp in a vegetable steamer over boiling water. Cover the pot and steam no more than 2 minutes. Remove pot from the heat and take off the lid to let the steam escape. Cover the pot again and let stand 3 to 4 minutes so shrimp can cook from the heat inside the shells. To remove the shells, push with your thumb and forefinger.

It is not necessary to devein the shrimp, but some people prefer it that way. (To devein shrimp, cut with a sharp-pointed knife along the outside curve of the body, remove the black vein.)

If desired, butter may be melted and dripped over shrimp. Otherwise, shrimp may be served as is, added to salads, or dressed with lemon, garlic, soy sauce, and herbs.

Yield: 1 serving

Five-spice Noodles with Chick-peas

2/3 cup chick-peas, rinsed and
  drained
1 cup (for women) or 1 1/2
  cups (for men) cooked pasta
1 large ripe tomato
1 stalk broccoli
2/3 cup canola oil

1/4 cup tarragon vinegar
1/2 teaspoon dried thyme
1/2 teaspoon dried marjoram
1/4 teaspoon black pepper
1/4 cup snipped fresh parsley
1/4 cup snipped fresh chives

Rinse canned chick-peas in a strainer and let drain. Prepare pasta according to instructions on page 104.

Wash tomato. Cut out stems. Slice lengthwise into quarters and cut quarters into 1/2-inch chunks. Wash and slice broccoli and steam in a vegetable steamer over boiling water for 5 minutes. Add tomato chunks to the steamer basket and steam for 5 more minutes.

Combine oil, vinegar, and herbs in a jar. Cover and shake well.

Combine chick-peas, pasta, and broccoli. Toss gently with 1 tablespoon herbed dressing for women or 2 tablespoons for men.

Yield: 3 1/2 cups for women, or 4 cups for men

Chicken-Shallot Sauté

3 ounces chicken, skin removed
1 tablespoon olive oil

1 large green bell pepper
4 shallots, chopped

Cut chicken into cubes. In a medium-sized frying pan over medium-high heat, brown chicken in olive oil. Seed the green pepper and cut it into julienne strips. Add pepper and shallots to chicken and sauté for 2 to 3 minutes over medium heat. Cover chicken and cook until tender (about 2 more minutes)

Yield: 1 serving

Potato Salad

1 small (3-ounce) potato, well
  scrubbed
1 cup green peas
2 cups of combined raw

carrots, celery, and onion
1 tablespoon Curry Dressing
  (see page 105)

Steam potato for 15 to 20 minutes. Add green peas and steam until tender, about 5 minutes more. Meanwhile, slice carrots, celery, and onion. When potato is cool enough to handle, cut into 1/2 inch cubes.

Combine all ingredients and toss with 1 tablespoon Curry Dressing or any dressing of your choice.

Yield: 1 serving

Sautéed Turkey with Asparagus and Pea Pods

4 ounces turkey breast, skin
  removed
1 tablespoon olive oil
1 tablespoon soy sauce

4 stalks asparagus, in 1/2-inch
  pieces
8 pea pods

Cut turkey breast into cubes. In a medium-sized frying pan over medium-high heat, brown the turkey in olive oil and soy sauce. Add asparagus and pea pods to turkey and sauté over medium heat for 2 to 3 minutes. Cover turkey and cook until tender, about 2 minutes more.

Yield: 1 serving

2. Using the blank menu plans on page 133, and keeping your own tastes and life-style in mind, allocate the exchanges in the blocks reserved for each meal.

3. Using the exchange lists on pages 134–142, choose the foods you wish to eat each day.

On the next pages, we give examples of allocation of food categories for the men's and women's high and low days. You needn't follow our recommendations exactly, but be sure to have at least three meals and two snacks every day, to encourage dietary-induced thermogenesis all day long.

After you have been on the Princeton Eating Plan for a while, the selection of foods should take little time and thought, and you may not even need to write down your menus. When you first begin planning, however, you may want to make several photocopies of the blank menu plans printed on page 133.

TABLE OF EXCHANGES FOR MEN'S AND WOMEN'S PRINCETON ALTERNATING EATING PLAN

	Milk	Veg	Fruit	Bread	Meat	Fat
Low-calorie, low-carbohydrate day						
Men: 1200 Calories	1	3	2	5	7	4
Women: 1000 Calories	1	3	2	3	6	4
High-calorie, high-carbohydrate day						
Men: 1700 Calories	2	4	4	12	0	7
Women: 1400 Calories	2	3	3	10	0	6

YOUR PERSONAL
EATING PLAN

NOW that you have followed our prepared menus for the Princeton Eating Plan, you may want to start creating your own menus from the wide variety of recommended foods. Your personal menus will continue to follow the Princeton guidelines, promoting maximum thermogenesis by alternating low-calorie, low-carbohydrate days with high-calorie, high-carbohydrate days, but you needn't worry about counting calories or figuring out carbohydrate percentages; that is taken care of automatically in the menu plans and exchange lists.

An *exchange* is a portion of food that is equivalent nutritionally to a portion of another food of the same type. For example, one small apple is equivalent to fifteen small grapes or ⅓ cup of cranberry juice. Each of these servings counts as one fruit exchange.

In using the exchange lists, think of foods as being divided into six categories: milk, vegetables, fruit, bread (which includes grains, pasta, and starchy vegetables), meat, and fat.

To use the exchange lists and plan your daily menu:

1. From the chart on page 128, determine how many exchanges of each type of food are allowed for the day.

Sample Menu Plan by Food Exchanges
Men's Low-Calorie, Low-Carbohydrate Day
1200 Calories

Breakfast 1 bread exchange 1 fat exchange 1/2 fruit exchange 1/2 milk exchange	**Morning Snack** 1 bread exchange 1/2 fruit exchange
Lunch 3 1/2 meat exchanges 1 1/2 bread exchanges 1 1/2 veg exchanges 1 1/2 fat exchanges	**Afternoon Snack** 1/2 fruit exchange
Dinner 3 1/2 meat exchanges 1 1/2 bread exchanges 1 1/2 veg exchanges 1 1/2 fat exchanges	**Evening Snack** 1/2 fruit exchange 1/2 milk exchange

Milk	Veg	Fruit	Bread	Meat	Fat
1	3	2	5	7	4

Sample Menu Plan by Food Exchanges
Men's High-Calorie, High-Carbohydrate Day
1700 Calories

Breakfast 2 1/2 bread exchanges 1 1/2 fat exchanges 1 fruit exchange 1 milk exchange	**Morning Snack** 2 1/2 bread exchanges 1 fruit exchange
Lunch 3 1/2 bread exchanges 2 veg exchanges 2 1/2 fat exchanges	**Afternoon Snack** 1 fruit exchange
Dinner 3 1/2 bread exchanges 2 veg exchanges 3 fat exchanges	**Evening Snack** 1 fruit exchange 1 milk exchange

Milk	Veg	Fruit	Bread	Meat	Fat
2	4	4	12	0	7

Sample Menu Plan by Food Exchanges
Women's Low-Calorie, Low-Carbohydrate Day
1000 Calories

Breakfast	Morning Snack
1/2 bread exchange 1 fat exchange 1/2 fruit exchange 1/2 milk exchange	1/2 bread exchange 1/2 fruit exchange
Lunch	**Afternoon Snack**
3 meat exchanges 1 bread exchange 1 1/2 veg exchanges 1 1/2 fat exchanges	1/2 fruit exchange
Dinner	**Evening Snack**
3 meat exchanges 1 bread exchange 1 1/2 veg exchanges 1 1/2 fat exchanges	1/2 fruit exchange 1/2 milk exchange

Milk	Veg	Fruit	Bread	Meat	Fat
1	3	2	3	6	4

Sample Menu Plan by Food Exchanges
Women's High-Calorie, High-Carbohydrate Day
1400 Calories

Breakfast 　　2 bread exchanges 　　1 fat exchange 　　½ fruit exchange 　　1 milk exchange	**Morning Snack** 　　2 bread exchanges 　　½ fruit exchange
Lunch 　　3 bread exchanges 　　1½ veg exchanges 　　2½ fat exchanges	**Afternoon Snack** 　　1 fruit exchange
Dinner 　　3 bread exchanges 　　1½ veg exchanges 　　2½ fat exchanges	**Evening Snack** 　　1 fruit exchange 　　1 milk exchange

Milk	Veg	Fruit	Bread	Meat	Fat
2	3	3	10	0	6

Low-Calorie, Low-Carbohydrate Menu Plan

Breakfast	Morning Snack
Lunch	Afternoon Snack
Dinner	Evening Snack

High-Calorie, High-Carbohydrate Menu Plan

Breakfast	Morning Snack
Lunch	Afternoon Snack
Dinner	Evening Snack

EXCHANGE LISTS

1. GRAIN/STARCH/PASTA/BREAD LIST

Each item contains 15 grams carbohydrate, 3 grams protein, a trace of fat, and 80 calories. If you want to eat a starch/bread food that is not on this list, the general rule is: ½ cup prepared grain, cereal, or pasta is 1 serving; 1 ounce of a bread product is 1 serving. Unless otherwise specified, amounts below are for the ready-to-eat form of the food.

Cereals/Grains/Pasta

Bran cereals, concentrated (Bran Buds, All Bran)	⅓ cup
Bran cereals, flaked	½ cup
Bulgur (cooked)	½ cup
Cooked cereals	½ cup
Cornmeal (dry)	2½ tablespoons
Grapenuts	3 tablespoons
Grits (cooked)	½ cup
Other ready-to-eat unsweetened cereals	¾ cup
Pasta (cooked)	½ cup
Puffed cereal	1½ cups
Rice, white or brown (cooked)	⅓ cup
Shredded wheat	½ cup
Wheat germ	3 tablespoons

Bread

Bagel	½ (1 ounce)
Breadsticks, crisp, 4 by ½ inch	2 (⅔ ounce)
Croutons, low-fat	1 cup
English muffin	½
Frankfurter or hamburger bun	½ (1 ounce)
Pita, 6 inches across	½
Plain roll, small	1 (1 ounce)
Raisin bread, unfrosted	1 slice
Rye or pumpernickel bread	1 slice
Tortilla, 6 inches across	1
Whole-wheat bread	1 slice

Dried Beans/Peas/Lentils

Baked beans (cooked)	1/4 cup
Beans and peas (cooked): kidney, navy, split, black-eyed, etc.	1/3 cup
Lentils (cooked)	1/3 cup

Starchy Vegetables

Corn	1/2 cup
Corn on cob, 6 inches long	1
Lima beans	1/2 cup
Peas, green (canned, frozen, or fresh)	1/2 cup
Plantain	1/2 cup
Potato, baked	1 small (3 ounces)
Potato, mashed	1/2 cup
Squash, winter (acorn, butternut)	3/4 cup
Yam, sweet potato, plain	1/3 cup

Crackers/Snacks

Crisp breads (Finn, Wasa)	2–4 crackers
Melba toast	5 slices
Popcorn, popped, no fat added	3 cups
Pretzels, whole-wheat	3/4 ounce
Rye crisp, 2 by 3 1/2 inches	4
Whole-wheat crackers (no fat added)	2–4 crackers

Starchy Foods Prepared with Fat (count as 1 starch plus 1 fat serving)

Biscuit, 2 1/2 inches across	1
Corn bread, 2-inch cube	1
Muffin, plain, small	1
Pancake, 4 inches across	2
Taco shell, 6 inches across	2

2. MEAT LIST

Each serving of meat or substitute on this list contains 7 grams protein. The fat and calorie content vary depending on whether the meat is lean, medium-fat, or high-fat. Please note the following equivalencies:

1 ounce meat = 1 meat exchange

4 ounces raw meat = 3 ounces cooked meat

2 ounces meat = 1 small chicken leg or thigh; 1/2 cup cottage cheese or tuna

3 ounces meat = 1 medium pork chop, 1 small hamburger, 1/2 whole chicken breast, 1 unbreaded fish fillet.

Lean Meat and Substitutes

One exchange is equal to any one of the following items and contains approximately 7 grams protein, 3 grams fat, and 55 calories.

Beef:	USDA Good or Choice grades of lean beef, such as round, sirloin, and flank steak; tenderloin; chipped beef	1 ounce
Pork:	Lean pork, such as fresh ham; canned, cured or boiled ham; Canadian bacon, tenderloin	1 ounce
Veal:	All cuts are lean except for veal cutlets (ground or cubed); examples of lean veal are chops and roasts	1 ounce
Poultry:	Chicken, turkey, Cornish hen (without skin)	1 ounce
Fish:	All fresh and frozen fish	1 ounce
	Crab, lobster, scallops, shrimp, clams (fresh or canned in water)	2 ounces
	Oysters	6 medium
	Tuna (canned in water)	1/4 cup
	Herring (uncreamed or smoked)	1 ounce
	Sardines (canned)	2 medium
Wild Game:	Venison, rabbit, squirrel	1 ounce
	Pheasant, duck, goose (without skin)	1 ounce
Cheese:	Cottage cheese, low-fat	1/4 cup
	Grated Parmesan	2 tablespoons
	Diet cheese (fewer than 55 calories/oz.)	1 ounce
	Lifetime-Brand cheeses	

Borden Lite-Line American and
Sharp Cheddar

| *Other:* | 95 percent fat-free luncheon meat | 1 ounce |
| | Egg whites | 3 |

Medium-Fat Meat and Substitutes

One exchange is equal to any one of the following items and contains approximately 7 grams protein, 5 grams fat, and 75 calories.

Beef:	Most beef products fall into this category. Examples are all ground beef, roast (rib, chuck, rump), steak, (cubed, porterhouse, T-bone), and meatloaf	1 ounce
Pork:	Most pork products fall into this category. Examples are chops, loin roast, Boston butt, cutlets	1 ounce
Lamb:	Most lamb products fall into this category. Examples are chops, leg, and roast	1 ounce
Veal:	Cutlet (ground or cubed, unbreaded)	1 ounce
Poultry:	Chicken (with skin), domestic duck or goose (well-drained of fat), ground turkey	1 ounce
Fish:	Tuna (canned in oil and drained) or salmon (canned)	¼ cup
Cheese:	Skim or part-skim milk cheeses such as,	
	Ricotta	¼ cup
	Mozzarella	1 ounce
	Diet cheeses (with 56–80 calories/oz.)	1 ounce
	Kraft Light Natural Swiss	
	Kraft Light 'n' Lively	
Other:	86 percent fat-free luncheon meat	1 ounce
	Whole egg	1

Tofu (2½- by 2¾- by 1-inch piece)   1 ounce
Liver, heart, kidney, sweetbreads   1 ounce

High-Fat Meats and Substitutes

One exchange is equal to any one of the following items and contains approximately 7 grams protein, 8 grams fat, and 100 calories. *With the exception of the nut butters,* these items should generally be avoided.

Beef:	Most USDA Prime cuts of beef, such as ribs, corned beef	1 ounce
Pork:	Spareribs, ground pork, pork sausage (patty or link)	1 ounce
Lamb:	Patties (ground lamb)	1 ounce
Fish:	Any fried-fish product	1 ounce
Cheese:	All regular cheeses, such as American, blue, Cheddar, Monterey Jack, Swiss	1 ounce
Other:	Luncheon meat, such as bologna, salami, pimento loaf	1 ounce
	Sausage, such as Polish, Italian	1 ounce
	Knockwurst, smoked	1 ounce
	Bratwurst	1 ounce
	Frankfurter (turkey or chicken)	1 frank (10/pound)
	Peanut, almond, cashew, and sunflower-seed butters (contain unsaturated fat)	1 tablespoon

(Count as 1 high-fat meat plus 1 fat exchange):

	Frankfurter (beef, pork, or combination)	1 frank (10/pound)

3. VEGETABLE LIST

One exchange is equal to 5 grams carbohydrate, 2 grams protein, and 25 calories. Unless otherwise noted, one vegetable exchange is: ½ cup cooked vegetables or vegetable juice; 1 cup raw vegetables.

Vegetables

Artichoke (½ medium)

Asparagus

Beans (green, wax, Italian)

Bean sprouts

Beets

Broccoli, broccoli rabe

Brussels sprouts

Cabbage, cooked, all kinds

Carrots

Cauliflower

Celery

Cucumbers

Eggplant

Greens (beet, chard, collard,
   dandelion)

Kale, mustard

Kohlrabi

Leeks

Mushrooms, cooked

Okra

Onions

Pea pods

Peppers (green, red, Italian)

Radicchio

Rutabaga

Sauerkraut

Spinach, cooked

Summer squash (crookneck)

Tomato (one large)

Tomato or vegetable juice

Turnips

Water chestnuts

Zucchini, cooked

Starchy vegetables such as corn, peas, potatoes, and winter squash are found on the Grain/Starch/Pasta/Bread List.

Free Vegetables (may be eaten as desired)

Chicory

Chinese cabbage

Endive

Escarole

Lettuce (all kinds: Boston,
   iceberg, romaine, etc.)

Parsley

Radishes

Watercress

4. MILK LIST

Each item contains about 12 grams carbohydrate and 8 grams protein. The fat and calories vary depending on what kind of milk you choose. Skim and very low-fat milks contain a trace of fat and 90 calories per cup. Low-fat milks contain 5 grams fat and 120 calories per cup.

Skim and Very Low-fat Milk

Skim milk	1 cup
1/2 percent milk	1 cup
1 percent milk	1 cup
Low-fat buttermilk	1 cup
Evaporated skim milk	1/3 cup
Dry nonfat milk	1/3 cup
Plain nonfat yogurt	1 cup

Low-fat Milk

2 percent milk	1 cup
Plain low-fat yogurt (with added nonfat milk solids)	1 cup

Cheese: see Meat List, page 135.

5. FRUIT LIST

Each item on this list contains about 15 grams carbohydrate and 60 calories. Unless otherwise noted, the serving size for one fruit serving is: 1/2 cup of fresh fruit or fruit juice; 1/4 cup of dried fruit.

Fresh, Frozen, and Unsweetened Canned Fruit

Apple, raw	1/2
Applesauce (unsweetened)	1/2 cup
Apricots (medium, raw)	4
Apricots (canned)	1/2 cup
Banana (9 inches long)	1/2
Blackberries (raw)	3/4 cup
Cantaloupe (5 inches across)	1/3 melon
cubes	1 cup
Cherries (large, raw)	12
Cherries (canned)	1/2 cup
Figs (raw, 2 inches across)	2
Fruit cocktail (canned)	1/2 cup
Grapefruit (medium)	1/2
Grapefruit (segments)	3/4 cup
Grapes (small)	15

Honeydew melon (medium)	1/8 melon
cubes	1 cup
Kiwi (large)	1
Mandarin oranges	3/4 cup
Mango (small)	1/2
Nectarine (1 1/2 inches across)	1
Orange (2 1/2 inches across)	1
Papaya	1 cup
Peach (2 3/4 inches across)	1
Peaches (canned)	1/2 cup (2 halves)
Pear (large)	1/2
(small)	1
Pears (canned)	1/2 cup (2 halves)
Persimmon (medium, native)	2
Pineapple (raw)	3/4 cup
Pineapple (canned)	1/3 cup
Plum (raw, 2 inches across)	2
Pomegranate	1/2
Raspberries (raw)	1 cup
Strawberries (raw, whole)	1 1/4 cups
Tangerine (2 1/2 inches across)	2
Watermelon (cubes)	1 1/4 cups

Dried Fruit

Apples	4 rings
Apricots	7 halves
Dates (medium)	2 1/2
Figs	1 1/2
Prunes (medium)	3
Raisins	2 tablespoons

Fruit Juice

Apple juice/cider	1/2 cup
Cranberry juice	1/3 cup
Grapefruit juice	1/2 cup
Grape juice	1/3 cup
Orange juice	1/2 cup
Pineapple juice	1/2 cup
Prune juice	1/3 cup

6. FAT LIST

Each serving on the fat list contains 5 grams fat and 45 calories.

Unsaturated Fats

Avocado	⅛ medium
Mayonnaise, nonhydrogenated	1 teaspoon
Mayonnaise, reduced-calorie	1 tablespoon
Oil (corn, cottonseed, safflower, soybean, sunflower, olive, peanut, walnut)	1 teaspoon
Salad dressing, mayonnaise-type	2 teaspoons
Salad dressing, mayonnaise-type, reduced-calorie	1 tablespoon
Salad dressing, all other varieties	1 tablespoon
Salad dressing, reduced-calorie	2 tablespoons

Saturated Fats

Bacon	1 slice
Butter	1 teaspoon
Chitterlings	½ ounce
Coconut, shredded	2 tablespoons
Cream cheese	1 tablespoon
Cream, light	2 tablespoons
Cream, sour	2 tablespoons
Cream, heavy	1 tablespoon
Nuts and Seeds	
Almonds	6 whole
Cashews	1 tablespoon
Peanuts	20 small or 10 large
Pecans	2 whole
Pine nuts	1 tablespoon
Walnuts	2 whole
Other nuts	1 tablespoon
Pumpkin seeds	2 teaspoons
Sunflower seeds (no shells)	1 tablespoon
Olives, green or black	10 small or 5 large
Salt pork	¼ ounce

FINE-TUNING THE PLAN

Our basic plan, with a "core" number of 1500 calories for men and 1200 for women, should enable most people to lose weight steadily. Not everyone is alike, however, and you may find that you need to alternate your daily calories around a higher or lower core figure. For example, if you are very overweight or have "yo-yoed" up and down many times, you may need to choose a lower core number than 1500 or 1200. If, on the other hand, you are very active, you may be more comfortable and satisfied with a higher core number.

For complete instructions on planning your own menus around a lower or higher core number of calories, please see Appendix A.

THE SIX-DAY
ROTATION PLAN

THIS chapter offers a variation on the Princeton Eating Plan for the convenience of those who travel or who eat frequently in restaurants, as well as for readers who don't want to plan their own menus. Unlike the Two-Week Plan, which offers as much variety as possible, the Six-Day Plan is predictable. For example, the high-carbohydrate breakfast is always cereal or pancakes, while all midday snacks consist of sunflower seeds and fruit. This uniformity means that any meal of a given type (e.g., a low-carbohydrate lunch) is interchangeable with the two other meals of that same type.

Please note that we have included a table of exchanges allowed for the Six-Day Plan so that you can make modifications to your own taste. Note also that the exchange tables are not identical to the exchange tables for the personalized Plan in chapter 10; the nutrient content is essentially the same, but different combinations of exchanges are used in each plan.

On pages 152 and 153 are blank charts developed by one of our clients to aid in keeping track of each day's foods.

FOOD EXCHANGES FOR SIX-DAY
ALTERNATING PLAN

Low-Calorie,
Low-Carbohydrate Days
Men
1200 calories
Breakfast:
  1 milk
  2 breads
  1 meat
Snack:
  1 fruit
Lunch:
  1 vegetable
  2 breads
  2 meats
  1 fat
Snack:
  1 fruit
  1 fat
Dinner:
  2 vegetables
  2 fats
  4 meats
Snack:
  1 fruit

Total:
  1 milk
  3 vegetables
  3 fruits
  4 breads
  4 fats
  7 meats

High-Calorie,
High-Carbohydrate Days
Men
1700 calories
Breakfast:
  1 milk
  3 breads
  2 fats
Snack:
  1 fruit
Lunch:
  2 vegetables
  3 breads
  2 fats
Snack:
  1 fruit
  1 fat
Dinner:
  6 breads
  2 vegetables
  3 fats
Snack:
  1 fruit
  1 milk

Total:
  2 milk
  4 vegetables
  3 fruits
  12 breads
  8 fats

FOOD EXCHANGES FOR SIX-DAY
ALTERNATING PLAN

Low-Calorie, Low-Carbohydrate Days Women 1000 calories	High-Calorie, High-Carbohydrate Days Women 1400 calories
Breakfast:	*Breakfast:*
1 milk	1 milk
1 bread	2 breads
1 meat	1 fat
Snack:	*Snack:*
1 fruit	1 fruit
Lunch:	*Lunch:*
1 vegetable	2 vegetables
2 breads	2 breads
2 meats	2 fats
Snack:	*Snack:*
1 fruit	1 fruit
1 fat	1 fat
Dinner:	*Dinner:*
2 vegetables	5 breads
2 fats	2 vegetables
3 meats	2 fats
Snack:	*Snack:*
1 fruit	1 fruit
	1 milk
Total:	*Total:*
1 milk	2 milk
3 vegetables	4 vegetables
3 fruits	3 fruits
3 breads	9 breads
3 fats	6 fats
6 meats	

THE PRINCETON SIX-DAY ROTATION PLAN FOR WOMEN

Day 1 LC/LC	Day 2 HC/HC	Day 3 LC/LC

Breakfast
Omelet
1 medium egg
1 cup skim milk
1 slice whole-grain
   bread
	Breakfast
	Cold Cereal
	1 cup flaked
	   whole-grain cereal
	1 cup skim milk
	1 tablespoon chopped
	   nuts
		Breakfast
		Cheese
		1 ounce low-fat cheese
		½ bagel
		1 cup skim milk

Snack 1 orange	**Snack** ½ grapefruit	**Snack** 1 orange

Lunch
Burger
2-ounce lean-beef
   burger
1 whole-grain roll
Lettuce
1 large tomato
	Lunch
	Veggie Pasta Salad
	1 cup steamed veggies
	1 cup cooked pasta
	2 tablespoons dressing
		Lunch
		Fish Sandwich
		½ cup tuna fish
		2 slices whole-grain
		   bread
		Veggies: 1 cup raw or
		   ½ cup steamed

Snack
1 fruit
1 tablespoon sunflower
   seeds
	Snack
	1 fruit
	1 tablespoon sunflower
	   seeds
		Snack
		1 fruit
		1 tablespoon sunflower
		   seeds

Dinner
Baked Fish
3 ounces bluefish
½ cup steamed green
   beans
1 teaspoon butter
1 green salad or 1
   small cucumber
1 tablespoon dressing
	Dinner
	Tamale
	⅔ cup cooked kidney
	   or pinto beans
	½ cup cooked corn
	1 cup cooked veggies:
	   onion, celery,
	   tomato, pepper
	Herbs (Hot red
	   pepper)
	2 teaspoons oil
	2 slices whole-grain
	   bread
		Dinner
		Stir-Fry Beef
		3 ounces meat (lean
		   beef, pork, lamb)
		2 cups raw veggies
		2 tablespoons oil

Snack 1 fruit	**Snack** 1 fruit 1 cup plain low-fat yogurt	**Snack** 1 fruit

THE PRINCETON SIX-DAY ROTATION PLAN FOR WOMEN

Day 4 HC/HC	Day 5 LC/LC	Day 6 HC/HC
Breakfast *Hot Cereal* 1 cup cooked oatmeal 1 cup skim milk 1 teaspoon butter	**Breakfast** *French Toast* 1 medium egg 1 cup skim milk 1 slice whole-grain bread	**Breakfast** *Pancakes* 4 pancakes, 4″ across 1 cup skim milk 2 teaspoons sugar-free jam or jelly
Snack ½ grapefruit	**Snack** 1 orange	**Snack** ½ grapefruit
Lunch *Potato-Veggie Salad* 1 6-ounce baked potato ½ cup green peas Veggies: 1 cup raw or ½ cup cooked 2 tablespoons dressing	**Lunch** *Poultry Sandwich* 2 ounces chicken/turkey 2 slices whole-grain bread Lettuce and tomato	**Lunch** *Veggie Pasta Salad* 1 cup steamed veggies 1 cup cooked pasta 2 tablespoons dressing
Snack 1 fruit 1 tablespoon sunflower seeds	**Snack** 1 fruit 1 tablespoon sunflower seeds	**Snack** 1 fruit 1 tablespoon sunflower seeds
Dinner *Legumes* 1 cup cooked lentils 1 cup cooked veggies 1 pita bread 2 teaspoons butter	**Dinner** *Shellfish* 6 ounces shrimp 1 teaspoon butter Garlic and lemon 2 cups steamed veggies 1 tablespoon dressing	**Dinner** *Spanish Rice* 1 cup cooked rice 1 cup cooked veggies Herbs 2 tortillas, 6″ across 2 teaspoons oil
Snack 1 fruit 1 cup plain low-fat yogurt	**Snack** 1 fruit	**Snack** 1 fruit 1 cup plain low-fat yogurt

THE PRINCETON SIX-DAY ROTATION PLAN FOR MEN

Day 1 LC/LC	Day 2 HC/HC	Day 3 LC/LC

Breakfast
Omelet
1 medium egg
1 cup skim milk
2 slices whole-grain
  bread
	Breakfast
	Cold Cereal
	1 1/2 cups flaked
	  whole-grain cereal
	1 cup skim milk
	2 tablespoons chopped
	  nuts
		Breakfast
		Cheese
		1 ounce low-fat cheese
		1 bagel
		1 cup skim milk

Snack 1 orange	**Snack** 1/2 grapefruit	**Snack** 1 orange

Lunch
Burger
2-ounce lean-beef
  burger
1 whole-grain roll
Lettuce
1 large tomato
1 tablespoon dressing
	Lunch
	Veggie Pasta Salad
	1 cup steamed veggies
	1 1/2 cups cooked pasta
	2 tablespoons dressing
		Lunch
		Fish Sandwich
		1/2 cup tuna fish
		2 slices whole-grain
		  bread
		Veggies: 1 cup raw or
		  1/2 cup steamed
		1 tablespoon dressing

Snack
1 fruit
1 tablespoon sunflower
  seeds
	Snack
	1 fruit
	1 tablespoon sunflower
	  seeds
		Snack
		1 fruit
		1 tablespoon sunflower
		  seeds

Dinner
Baked Fish
4 ounces bluefish
1/2 cup steamed green
  beans
1 teaspoon butter
1 green salad or 1
  small cucumber
1 tablespoon dressing
	Dinner
	Tamale
	2/3 cup cooked kidney
	  or pinto beans
	1 cup cooked corn
	1 cup cooked veggies:
	  onion, celery,
	  tomato, pepper
	Herbs (Hot red
	  pepper)
	1 tablespoon oil
	2 slices whole-grain
	  bread
		Dinner
		Stir-Fry Beef
		4 ounces meat (lean
		  beef, pork, lamb)
		2 cups raw veggies
		2 tablespoons oil

Snack 1 fruit	**Snack** 1 fruit 1 cup plain low-fat yogurt	**Snack** 1 fruit

THE PRINCETON SIX-DAY ROTATION PLAN FOR MEN

Day 4 HC/HC	Day 5 LC/LC	Day 6 HC/HC

Breakfast
Hot Cereal
1 ½ cups cooked
  oatmeal
1 cup skim milk
2 teaspoons butter
	Breakfast
	French Toast
	1 medium egg
	1 cup skim milk
	2 slices whole-grain
	  bread
		Breakfast
		Pancakes
		6 pancakes, 4″ across
		1 cup skim milk
		2 teaspoons sugar-free
		  jam or jelly
		1 teaspoon butter

Snack ½ grapefruit	**Snack** 1 orange	**Snack** ½ grapefruit

Lunch
Potato-Veggie Salad
1 6-ounce baked
  potato
½ cup green peas
Veggies: 1 cup raw or
  ½ cup cooked
4 wheat crackers
2 tablespoons dressing
	Lunch
	Poultry Sandwich
	2 ounces
	  chicken/turkey
	2 slices whole-grain
	  bread
	Lettuce and tomato
	1 teaspoon mayonnaise
		Lunch
		Veggie Pasta Salad
		1 cup steamed veggies
		1 ½ cups cooked pasta
		2 tablespoons dressing

Snack
1 fruit
1 tablespoon sunflower
  seeds
	Snack
	1 fruit
	1 tablespoon sunflower
	  seeds
		Snack
		1 fruit
		1 tablespoon sunflower
		  seeds

Dinner *Legumes* 1 cup cooked lentils 1 cup cooked veggies 1 ½ pita breads 1 tablespoon butter	**Dinner** *Shellfish* 8 ounces shrimp 1 teaspoon butter Garlic and lemon 2 cups steamed veggies 1 tablespoon dressing	**Dinner** *Spanish Rice* 1 cup cooked rice 1 cup cooked veggies Herbs 3 tortillas, 6″ across 1 tablespoon oil

Snack
1 fruit
1 cup plain low-fat
  yogurt
	Snack
	1 fruit
		Snack
		1 fruit
		1 cup plain low-fat
		  yogurt

SAMPLE MENU CHARTS FOR PRINCETON
SIX-DAY ROTATION PLAN

Women, Week #

| | | | | 1000 | 1 | 3 | 3 | 3 | 6 | 3 |
| | | | | 1400 | 2 | 4 | 3 | 9 | 0 | 6 |

Breakfast	Lunch	Dinner	Snacks	Milk	Veg.	Fruit	Bread	Meat	Fat

SAMPLE MENU CHARTS FOR PRINCETON
SIX-DAY ROTATION PLAN

Men, Week #

Breakfast	Lunch	Dinner	Snacks	Milk	Veg.	Fruit	Bread	Meat	Fat
1200				1	3	3	4	7	4
1700				2	4	3	12	0	8

PART III

THE PRINCETON EXERCISE PLAN

BORN TO MOVE

IN Part I, we explained some of the reasons why exercise is a necessary part of any weight-loss plan. Exercise not only burns calories and increases metabolic rate; it also limits or even prevents the loss of muscle that usually occurs when weight is lost. The psychological benefits of exercise, which range from improved self-esteem to stress reduction, can also make it easier to stick with any new regimen.

Still, we realize that for many readers, especially those who have been sedentary for a long time, the idea of beginning an exercise program can be daunting—especially in an era where physical fitness is often equated with such strenuous activities as marathon running or the high-fashion world of aerobic dancing. **We'd like to reassure you that the Princeton Exercise Plan is well within the capabilities of even the most dedicated couch potato.** Our program consists of three parts, and you start each at the level that is right for you. As your physical condition improves, you may wish to progress further and practice at a more strenuous or even competitive level. But you needn't ever run so much as a one-block race or invest in any designer sweatbands or other trendy exercise gear. If you choose, in fact, you can do the entire three-part program in your pajamas, completely within the privacy of your own home.

In the next few chapters we will give you specific guidelines on performing a number of exercises, each of which has a specific purpose in the context of the overall Princeton Plan. But bear in mind as you read that **the main purpose of our exercise plan is to encourage you, no matter what your present level of fitness, to move more**. Our bodies were made for movement, and lack of movement contributes to excess weight and to degenerative conditions such as arthritis and the "stiffness" of old age. Remember that any amount of activity is good and adds to your store of fitness. Bear in mind also that the more overweight or sedentary you are now, the greater the potential benefits of any amount of exercise. An 800-pound man, for example, would begin to improve his fitness level just by getting out of bed.

An example of the dramatic results that can be achieved by even a small amount of exercise is provided by a seventy-two-year-old man we know. Like many men whose lives have been structured around their work, Frank became increasingly sedentary after he retired. Eventually, his long-standing diabetes became severe enough to require daily injections of insulin.

On his doctor's advice, Frank began to exercise, walking very slowly four to five blocks a day. To his amazement, even that seemingly insignificant amount of exercise made a big difference, enabling him to stabilize his blood sugar levels more easily and then gradually to reduce the amount of insulin he took daily. Of course, as Frank becomes even more fit he will need to increase his level of exercise, but his present improvement seems to him almost miraculous. "I never realized that such a tiny amount of exercise could make such a big difference," he says.

Frank's experience is not unique; a recent California study found that Frank's current level of exercise—walking only five blocks a day—reduced volunteers' risk of coronary heart disease by 21 percent; more vigorous activity conferred even greater benefits.

Are you ready to give it a try? You have nothing to lose—except excess weight—and everything to gain in health and well-being.

The first part of the Princeton Exercise Plan consists of **whole-body exercises**: running, swimming, walking, and the like. These are the exercises that increase thermogenesis and metabolism, reduce appetite, and reduce the risk for a number of diseases. You should do them at least three, and preferably four or five, times a week. The second part of the plan, performed three times a week, focuses on **strength-building exercises** to increase muscle mass, thus upping

WHOLE-BODY
EXERCISES: AEROBICS

WHAT IS FITNESS?

PHYSICAL fitness is synonymous with being "in shape." But what constitutes fitness for one person may very well be an inadequate level of fitness for another. For example, if you are a schoolteacher, fitness would include the stamina necessary to instruct in front of a class all day, as well as to participate in your regular daily activities. A Marine drill instructor, on the other hand, would need to be stronger and able to run several miles at a time. As defined by the President's Council on Physical Fitness, fitness is "the ability to carry out daily tasks with vigor and alertness . . . and with ample energy to enjoy leisure-time pursuits and to meet unusual situations and unforeseen emergencies." Fitness, in other words, is the ability to lead an active, effective, and enjoyable life.

Fitness is not, by the way, the same thing as health, which is defined by the World Health Organization as "a state of physical, mental, and social well-being and not merely the absence of disease and infirmity." It is possible to be very fit physically—like the late Jim Fixx, running guru and marathoner—and yet have a serious underlying disease. In your resting metabolic rate, as well as producing a leaner, firmer appearance. The third component of the plan consists of what we call **life-style exercises**—simple activities that you can easily incorporate into your daily routine to burn extra calories all day long.

Fixx's case, his fitness led him to believe that he was also healthy, and he ignored the warning signs of serious heart disease that led to his death while jogging. The ideal is to be both fit and healthy, a prime goal of the Princeton Plan.

Physiologists recognize a number of components of physical fitness: Among the most important are muscular strength and endurance, flexibility, and aerobic fitness. The first two measures are easy to determine—you probably have a pretty good idea right now how much you can lift and carry and how long it takes your arms to tire when you're carrying suitcases through an airport. Likewise, you probably already know whether you can touch your toes—a measure of flexibility.

Chances are, however, you do not know very much about your present level of aerobic fitness, which is a measure of the health of your heart, lungs, and circulatory system. In fact, when you hear the word "aerobics," you may, like many Americans, immediately think of a room full of young women in color-coordinated leotards and leg warmers, jumping and kicking to a disco beat. What you are visualizing is aerobic dance, which, though it is sometimes referred to as "aerobics," is only one of a wide variety of aerobic activities.

What all aerobic exercises have in common is that they promote the intake and use of oxygen, strengthening your heart, lungs, and circulatory system and improving the health of all your body systems. An exercise is aerobic if it is sustained and strenuous enough to raise your heartbeat and cause you to break out in a sweat but not so strenuous that you find yourself gasping for breath, your heart pounding furiously. This latter type of exercise is called **anaerobic**, meaning "without oxygen," and that gasping, exhausted feeling is the result of your body's inability to deliver an adequate supply of oxygen to the muscles. For most sedentary people, a brisk walk would be aerobic, while a sprint to catch a bus would be anaerobic, because during the run to the bus body tissues are receiving insufficient oxygen. For a trained athlete, however, both activities would be aerobic, as would a slow run of several miles.

Aerobic exercises build your stamina and endurance and quickly increase the capacity of your heart to deliver oxygenated blood throughout your body. Because they make your cardiovascular system more efficient, these exercises improve your endurance and at the same time give you more energy for anything you want to do. And they are essential when it comes to weight loss. **Research shows that the sustained nature of aerobic exercise prevents the metabolic slow-**

down caused by dieting, while increasing levels of the prostaglandins (PGE1 and PGE3) that stimulate brown fat. Aerobic exercise also helps move fat out of its stores in fatty tissue, making it more accessible for burning as fuel. In fact, studies show that the more conditioned (aerobically fit) you are, the greater your ability to burn fat each time you exercise.

Although the fat-burning capability conferred by aerobic exercise increases the longer the exercise session lasts, all that is needed to begin to make fat available for fuel is to perform at a steady, aerobic pace for 15 minutes. Long-distance runners and other endurance athletes have very low percentages of body fat because of their efficiency at burning fat stores.

Of course, following an aerobic exercise program will require some effort, like anything worthwhile. But you can significantly improve your own aerobic condition in as little as 30 minutes a day, three times a week. Even this level of aerobics will give you minimal aerobic fitness and help speed weight loss. However, for a significant increase in thermogenesis, exercise must be more frequent. To maximize your own weight loss, try to do at least a little aerobics five to six times a week.

WHICH EXERCISE IS BEST?

There are a wide variety of aerobic exercises, and one is sure to be right for you. Among the most popular are aerobic dance, walking, jogging, bicycling, swimming, cross-country skiing, and rowing. One of the best exercises for beginners is Dr. Heleniak's own **aerobic prancing**, which is an excellent, nonstressful exercise for anyone beginning exercise after years of sedentary living or anyone who is seriously overweight.

When planning your own aerobic program, choose something that you enjoy and that you can continue without inconveniencing yourself; otherwise you are building in failure. For example, if you choose swimming but you live 50 miles from the nearest swimming pool, you will need an almost superhuman level of commitment to continue the program. Likewise, if you are very overweight or suffer from arthritis or other joint disorders, you should probably choose a non-weight-bearing activity, such as bicycling or stationary bicycling, using a rowing machine, or swimming.

On pages 165–172 we give complete guidelines for a progressive walking/running program and for aerobic prancing. But if you prefer a different aerobic activity, that is fine. There are many excellent books available on all aerobic exercises; in addition, most Ys and health clubs offer classes for beginners. Whichever activity you choose, be sure to follow these guidelines:

1. *See your doctor before you begin any exercise program.* This is especially important for anyone who is overweight, older than thirty-five, or has a personal or family history of heart disease.

    Depending on your medical history, your doctor may want to give you an exercise stress test, in which he or she monitors the condition of your heart while you walk on a treadmill. We especially recommend such a test for anyone who has a personal or family history of heart disease.

    "I feel fine," you may think. "Why should I pay a doctor to tell me what I already know?" Such an attitude may be understandable and is unfortunately common, but it can be very dangerous. If you are tempted to go ahead with the plan without a doctor's okay, we urge you to remember Jim Fixx and think again! A number of supposedly very fit men and women have died of heart attacks while exercising—in most cases because they suffered from "hidden heart disease" and were exercising at a pace far too strenuous for their condition. Similarly, if, during exercise, you experience *any* feelings of pain or pressure in your chest, neck, or jaw, stop exercising immediately and consult your doctor.

    We don't mean to scare you. Exercise is completely safe for the vast majority of Americans, even those who are overweight. In fact, aerobic exercise can *improve* the health of your heart and is often used in a supervised setting in cardiac-rehabilitation programs. But it makes sense for you to know exactly where you stand and pace your training program accordingly.

2. *Start slowly.* This caveat applies both to each exercise session and to your exercise program as a whole. Especially if you are overweight and/or unused to physical activity, it is important to begin any program slowly and not to expect miracles. Re-

mind yourself that it has taken years to get out of shape; it will take at least a few months to get fit. Don't force yourself to do more than you are ready for, because pushing yourself too hard can lead to exhaustion and sore muscles and is one of the main reasons many people drop out of exercise programs before they have given the activity a fair chance.

3. *Make a time commitment.* Before you even begin your program, plan in advance *which* days you will be doing your aerobic exercise and *when.* Without a definite plan, you may find it easy to skip sessions and thus lose the benefits. (For a sample exercise and eating plan, see page 196.)

4. *Warm up before you begin.* No matter which aerobic exercise(s) you choose, it is important to spend a few minutes warming up your muscles and revving up your heartbeat. Just as you would not expect your car to start right up on a cold morning, so you should not expect your body to begin activity from a standing stop. The best warmup for any aerobic activity is simply to do that activity slowly, then gradually increase the pace. Thus, for a walking program, walk slowly for the first 5 minutes; for biking, bike slowly.

    After you have warmed up, you may want to stop and stretch before continuing—or you may enjoy the feel of stretching *after* the exercise. For more on stretching, a vital part of the third component of the Princeton Exercise Plan, see pages 191–193.

5. *Exercise within your training heart rate.* Your **training heart rate**, also sometimes called your **target heart range**, is the rate of heartbeats per minute that will strengthen your cardiovascular system and increase your aerobic fitness. It is not a fixed rate but rather a range that is determined by both your age and your present aerobic condition.

    The target rate is one at which your pulse is elevated, but not to the point where you can feel your heart "thudding" in your chest. A quick way to determine if you are working within your target range is to sing to yourself (or talk to a companion). If you can easily do so, without gasping, and yet you are still getting a noticeable workout, you are within your target range. As long as you're working hard enough to break out in a light sweat, you needn't ever determine your heart rate more precisely than that. But if you would like to know exactly what your target heart range is, use the following formula:

- Subtract your age from 220.
- Multiply the result by both .6 and .8.

These two numbers represent the lower and upper boundaries of your target heart range, respectively, and this is the range within which you should be working when you do your aerobic exercise.

To determine if you are working within your target range, immediately after stopping, take your pulse for 10 seconds and multiply it by 6, for heartbeats per minute. (The easiest place to find your pulse is at your carotid artery, toward the center of your neck, just under the jawline.)

As you become more aerobically fit, you will discover that the same amount of work no longer suffices to move your pulse into the target range and that you will have to exercise at a faster pace to achieve the same results. It's true that this means more work, but it's also tangible proof that your program is working!

6. *Cool down.* During the most strenuous phase of your aerobic workout, much of your body's blood supply is directed to your muscles, and your heart is beating well above its resting rate. To give your cardiovascular system a chance to return gradually to normal, don't stop your workout abruptly; rather, continue at a slower pace for at least 5 minutes.

BEGINNING A WALKING PROGRAM

Walking is probably the easiest and most practical aerobic exercise, because it can be done by virtually anyone, no matter how out of shape.

All you need to get started are a good pair of walking or jogging shoes and a place to walk.

CHOOSING SHOES

While it's true that generations of American men have marched millions of miles in stiff army boots, your feet will thank you if you get shoes made specifically for walking. If you think that you may want to progress to jogging, get running shoes, which are also just fine for walking.

Shoes made specifically for walking cushion and protect your feet in a way that old-fashioned generic tennis sneakers cannot. Although decent walking or jogging shoes are not cheap, you should be able to find something adequate for around $40. Try on the shoes with the socks you will be wearing (plain cotton or Orlon-cotton mix are best for sweat absorption), and walk around the store until you are sure that the shoes are comfortable.

DECIDING WHAT TO WEAR

When the fitness boom began back in the 1970s, most joggers wore baggy gray sweatpants and jackets because that was what was available. Today those same soft cotton sweats can still be found, but they now come in a rainbow of colors. There are also tights, leotards, and warmup suits, some designer styled or made of high-tech fabrics that adjust to different weather conditions.

If wearing such a space-age outfit will help put you in the exercise mood, and you can afford it, by all means invest in exercise clothes. But bear in mind that you needn't spend a penny; you undoubtedly have some old clothes around the house that would be perfect: comfortable slacks or jeans, a soft T-shirt or sweatshirt. You can walk in literally any sort of clothing; the best for exercise is an outfit that is loose enough to allow unrestricted movement, with no tight waistbands or cuffs that could cause discomfort or chafing. Absorbent materials—meaning cotton or wool—are best. You may prefer to walk in street clothes, especially if you're embarrassed about beginning an exercise program and don't want to call attention to yourself. On the other hand, a nun, who is frequently spotted jogging in New York City's Riverside Park, runs in her full habit (plus running shoes). In cold weather, dress in layers: Add a sweater, and/or a windbreaker, which you can remove and wrap around your waist if you begin to get too hot.

DECIDING WHERE TO WALK

One great advantage to choosing walking as your aerobic exercise is that it can literally be done anywhere. One caveat, though: It is best to chose a route where you will be able to walk continuously, without worrying about curbs and without having to stop frequently for traffic lights or pedestrian congestion. If you live in a city, a nearby park is usually the best place to follow your program.

In the suburbs, you have more leeway. You can walk in your neighborhood, or around a large structure, like a school. If you want to know exactly how far you have walked, travel the distance of the route in your car, noting the stopping and starting numbers on your odometer. Or walk on the track at a nearby school before or after school hours.

If you live in a large apartment building, you can walk in the halls of your building. Or check out the local mall. Growing numbers of malls all across the country are opening early for the convenience of health walkers. These covered arcades eliminate any excuses for skipping your workout, since they are protected in all weather conditions. Not only can you get your aerobic exercise in, you may make new friends at the same time.

DECIDING WHEN TO WALK

On page 196, we offer a sample schedule of alternating diet and exercise days.

What time of day you choose to do your walking depends on your own convenience and energy level. Early risers, for example, usually like to exercise first thing in the morning, while night people, not surprisingly, often find that a late-afternoon or early-evening exercise bout energizes them for an active evening. **No matter what time you choose to exercise, the most important thing is to schedule your aerobic session *before* one of the three major meals of the day, to** boost your metabolism, cut your appetite, and increase dietary-induced thermogenesis.

BUILDING A WALKING PROGRAM

The following program is designed for someone who is very over-weight and/or has been sedentary for many years. If you are in some-what better shape, then you can begin at a more advanced Stage. Remember that for aerobic fitness you must exercise at least three times a week; for more rapid weight loss, increase your workouts to five or six days a week.

Stage One. Walk 5 to 10 minutes, at any pace that is comfortable. If you need to stop and rest, do so, then continue. Continue at Stage One until your stamina has improved and you can walk comfortably and continuously for 10 minutes.

Stage Two. Add 5 minutes to your walk, until you can walk comfortably and continuously for 15 minutes.

Stage Three. Continue to extend your walk until you can walk comfortably and continuously for 20 minutes.

Stage Four. Continue to walk 20 minutes, but during the middle 10 minutes of your exercise session walk more briskly, so that your breathing is more rapid and you are perhaps beginning to perspire. *Do not* walk so briskly that you feel out of breath; you should be able to carry on a conversation or sing to yourself. If you wish, you can start taking your pulse to determine if you are in your target heart range (see page 164).

Stage Five. Extend the walk to 25 minutes. The first 5 and last 5 minutes of the walk should be relatively slow, while the remaining 15 minutes should be brisk.

Stage Six and *Maintenance.* Extend your walk to 30 minutes. Five minutes should be warmup, 20 minutes brisk walking in your target heart range, and 5 minutes at a slower walk to cool down.

Do not worry about how long it takes you to complete each Stage; that will depend entirely on your present condition and age. Do not go on to the next Stage until you have reached the goal of the present Stage.

When you have completed Stage Six, you may remain there, on maintenance. If you wish to continue increasing your fitness level beyond this Stage, then *gradually:*

1. increase your walking pace; or

2. carry light hand weights; or

3. begin to mix in jogging (see below).

BEGINNING A JOGGING PROGRAM

A regular walking program is all the aerobic exercise most people need. But you may find, as you become more fit, that you want to engage in more vigorous activity. If so, once you have completed Stage Six of the walking program, you can gradually switch to a more demanding aerobic program. The following guidelines are for converting your walking program to jogging.

In many respects, jogging is not very different from walking, but it is far harder on your feet, ankles, knees, and hips, so a pair of good jogging shoes is a *must.* Also, beware of the tendency, common among many people who have become fit after years of inactivity, to try to turn into an instant track star; continue to work at a pace that is comfortably within your target heart range.

Continue with Stage Six, but now begin to add in a few minutes of jogging to your 30 minutes of walking. Don't overdo; simply alternate jogging and walking during the middle 20 minutes of your program. Work up to a continuous 20-minute jog, preceded and followed by 5 minutes of walking.

DR. HELENIAK'S AEROBIC PRANCING

Aerobic prancing is one of the best of all aerobic exercises, especially for beginners, because it requires no previous experience and can be performed at any level of fitness. It is the ideal way to ease into an exercise regimen for the following reasons as well:

- Unlike dance aerobics and jogging, it is not stressful to the joints.

- It can be performed entirely in the privacy of your home and thus can be done in any kind of weather or even after dark.

- It requires no special clothing or equipment.

- Because it's done at home, you needn't worry about traffic, dogs, potholes, or inhaling automobile exhaust.

- Because you can watch TV or listen to music while exercising, it is less likely to get boring.

In many ways aerobic prancing resembles the movements of aerobic dance and low-impact aerobics, but because it is less programmed and relies less on dance moves, it can easily be performed even by someone with two left feet.

When you begin your aerobic prancing program, remember never to overdo—any movement is better than none.

Most aerobic prancers enjoy exercising to music, as it helps you perform rhythmically and also helps the time pass quickly.

1. *Place-Walk Warmup.* The first few minutes of your routine are a warmup to get your heart and muscles revved up and ready to go. Walk in place with your hands on your hips. As you become more warmed up, you may increase the pace of your steps and/or the height at which you step. When you are beginning, especially if you are very overweight or have been sedentary for a long time, you may do only the warmup. As it becomes easier, begin to add the other parts of the program.

2. *Side Slide.* Taking steps from side to side, move across the room or even from room to room. Swing your arms, or make big circles in the air with your hands. Remember that the idea is to use your body and move as much as possible.

3. *Retro-walk.* Walk backward, around the room, or from room to room. This movement helps strengthen the front muscles of your legs.

4. *Steps.* This move is the most strenuous and therefore the best for getting your heartbeat in your target range (see page 164–165); begin it only after you have worked up to at least 10 minutes of continuous prancing.

   If you have a two-step footstool or stairs, simply climb up and down the two steps in a rhythmic movement. When you first begin, go slowly, then gradually build up speed. If you don't have access to steps, try the following variant:

   Place a large, thick book (a phone book is ideal) or a block of wood on the floor. In a rhythmic movement, step on it with your right foot, then your left, so you are standing with all your weight on the book. Pause momentarily, then step off, one foot at a time. Repeat, in a rhythmic movement, for up to 5 minutes.

5. *Figure Eights.* Walking forward three or four steps, and then back the same amount, create one or more "figure eights" or other patterns.

6. *Imaginary Rope.* Pretend that you are jumping rope for several beats (don't forget to use your arms to "turn" the imaginary rope).

Practice combining the different parts of the program, until you can "prance" for 30 full minutes. You needn't do the different steps in any particular order, except for the warmup and cool down.

1. Place-Walk: Warmup

2. Side Slide

3. Steps

4. Figure Eights

5. Imaginary Rope

6. Side Slide

7. Steps

8. Retro-walk

9. Place-Walk Cool Down

ADVANCED PRANCING

When you can "prance" comfortably and continuously for 30 minutes, you may wish to add the following elements to make the routine more challenging:

1. Begin "Steps" on a low stool or chair.

2. Do parts of the routine faster.

3. Mix in vigorous dance steps. Especially good are the Irish jig, polka, and hora; less vigorous but still good exercise are the cha-cha, waltz, and fox-trot.

You may also wish, at this point, to begin a more structured exercise program. There are a number of excellent videotapes on low-impact aerobics. If you wish to begin a walking or jogging program, see pages 165–170.

MUSCLE BUILDERS

ALTHOUGH regular aerobic exercise is the key to revving up metabolism and improving overall health, strength-building exercises are a must in any weight-loss program. This is so for two reasons.

First, as we explained in Part I, muscle tissue is more active metabolically than fat tissue; that is, it requires more energy simply to maintain itself. Thus, the higher the ratio of muscle to fat in your body, the higher your resting metabolism rate (RMR).

Second, muscle tissue is denser than fat; it weighs more but takes up less space. Thus, as you replace fat with muscle you will dramatically lose inches, even though you may not be losing pounds as quickly as you'd like.

Good muscle strength and tone confer other benefits as well; among them are better posture, which also improves appearance, and more stamina for doing the things you want to do all day long. If you enjoy any sort of recreational sport, you will probably find that your skill level improves as you become stronger. For women a strength-building program is especially beneficial, since most women are severely deficient in upper-body strength. This relative weakness often causes problems in daily life, ranging from difficulty in lifting and carrying to deterioration of posture, exacerbation of "dowager's hump," and back problems. Following a systematic program to build upper-body strength can improve your appearance, and will also help eliminate back pain and make it easier to perform such troublesome tasks as moving furniture or even opening stuck jars without help.

There is no danger, by the way, that a woman following our program will become "muscle bound"—most women do not possess sufficient levels of testosterone, the male hormone responsible for large muscle size.

WHAT MAKES A MUSCLE GROW?

Just as your cardiovascular system responds to aerobic exercise by becoming stronger, so your muscles, when they are challenged, respond by growing stronger to handle the challenge. On a physiological level, the muscle fibers themselves change, increasing their ability to use energy to produce movement. Although exercise cannot change the number of muscle fibers, each individual fiber grows larger.

There are three methods of challenging your muscles and causing them to grow stronger; each of these is based on the principle known as **progressive resistance**. *Resistance* is the challenge your muscles work against: their own tension, gravity, or a weight. In order to make your muscles stronger, you must *progressively* increase the resistance that you ask them to work against.

To see how this works in practice, suppose you carry a 10-pound briefcase home from the bus stop every day. Then you get a new portable computer that weighs 3 pounds, increasing the weight you are used to carrying to 13 pounds. You will probably find it difficult to lug this new weight home and may even have to stop and rest on the way. But in a very few days you will notice that it becomes easier to carry the extra weight; after a week or two it will be as easy as it had been to carry the old lighter briefcase.

What has happened is that your muscles, challenged by the extra weight, have responded by becoming bigger and stronger. And it is this ability of your muscles that makes systematic strength-building exercises possible.

Returning to the briefcase analogy, if you wanted to improve your briefcase-toting ability even further, you might try adding a 1-pound book every few days or carrying the briefcase a few steps farther each evening. Although the added challenge would be difficult to meet at first, your muscles would quickly respond with increased strength.

There are three types of strength-building exercises that make use of progressive resistance. These are **isotonic, isokinetic,** and **isometric** exercises.

Isotonic exercises are any exercises in which you *move* a muscle. The most familiar examples are weight lifting and calisthenics, but actually most of your daily activities, from lifting a cup of coffee to dialing the telephone, are examples of isotonic exercises. In each case the muscles involved contract and extend through a range of motion against a resistance (gravity, the telephone, the weight of your own body).

Isokinetic exercises are a form of weight training, done on special machines that provide a variable resistance as the muscle moves through its whole range of motion.

Isometric exercises are those in which the muscle *contracts* but does not *move.* Closing your fist tightly and holding it is an example of an isometric exercise.

Any of these three types of exercise can be used to strengthen muscles and increase muscle mass. The best-known is probably weight training, which can be done either with freestanding weights (barbells and dumbbells) or machines, such as Nautilus and Universal. These exercises must generally be performed in a gym or health club, both for access to the equipment and because expert supervision is necessary for proper technique and safety.

Isometric exercises, on the other hand, can be performed at home without supervision, take only a few minutes each week, and can dramatically increase muscular strength in a relatively short period of time.

Isometric exercises are not as good as isotonic or isokinetic exercises for increasing a muscle's strength throughout its entire range of motion, because an isometrically trained muscle is strongest in the position in which the contraction is performed. For maximum effectiveness, then, isometric exercises should be performed in several positions. Apart from this one caveat, these simple exercises have many advantages:

- **Isometrics quickly increase muscle mass.** In one experiment, a twelve-year-old volunteer greatly increased the amount of muscle in his right leg in only three weeks, by performing ten

10-second isometric contractions three times a week. Those old comic-book ads that promised to build big beautiful muscles on 120-pound weaklings worked on the same principle.

- **Isometrics minimize soreness and injury.** Studies have shown that while isometric exercises are as effective as isotonic exercises in increasing musculature, they are much less likely to cause injury or strain to muscles and joints and are less likely to cause muscle soreness.

- **Isometric exercises are fast and convenient.** Because they can be done at home and take less time than other strength-building exercises, isometrics are ideal for anyone whose time is limited or who is just starting to exercise and is reluctant to make too large a time commitment.

HOW TO DO ISOMETRIC EXERCISES

There is not enough room in this book to give guidelines for a strength-building program using free weights or machines. This is not to say that those exercises are inordinately difficult but merely that proper technique is essential for the desired results, and supervision is therefore important when you are beginning. If you wish to take up any of the various forms of weight training, "more power to you"; a growing number of Americans are finding that this form of exercise is the perfect complement to aerobics. (See the Selected Bibliography for a list of recommended books on weight training.)

Although certain guidelines must be followed for maximum benefit from isometric exercises, they are much easier to learn than isotonic exercises. Below are general guidelines for beginning your isometric program.

1. *Check with your doctor before beginning the Princeton Isometric Plan.* Although isometrics are for the most part very safe, they can be dangerous for people with high blood pressure and certain other vascular conditions. Unfortunately, high blood pressure does not usually have symptoms; therefore, see your doctor and get his or her okay before starting.

2. *Read through the instructions for all exercises before you begin the regimen,* so you will be certain how to perform them. Then, following the instructions, contract the muscle or muscles as tightly as you can and hold the contraction, at maximum strength. Unless otherwise noted, the muscles involved in each exercise should remain stationary, though you may notice a slight trembling in the muscle being exercised, especially when you are first getting used to the program. When you begin, hold each contraction for 1 to 3 seconds; as your muscles become stronger, work up to 7 seconds.

Unless otherwise stated in the instructions, you need to perform each contraction only once; if you wish, you may perform them more times for faster progress.

If you find it inconvenient to watch the second hand of a clock or watch while you are performing a contraction, you can get a rough estimate by counting slowly: "one thousand one," "one thousand two," etc. Each number represents approximately 1 second.

3. *Breathe naturally as you perform the contractions.* This may seem difficult at first, because the normal inclination when contracting muscles is to hold your breath.

4. *Don't overdo.* When you first begin performing the Princeton Isometric Plan, you may find it difficult to hold a contraction at full intensity. Just do the best you can, and, following the principle of progressive resistance, gradually work up to full 7-second contractions. One great benefit of resistance-training exercises is that you can often see results from one session to the next. As you are able to extend the amount of time and the force of the contractions, you will know you are building muscle and turning up your resting metabolism rate.

THE PRINCETON ISOMETRIC PROGRAM

The following isometric program consists of ten exercises, each designed to strengthen a different muscle group. Several of the exercises are performed in more than one position so that the muscle will become strengthened throughout a greater range of motion.

BICEPS PRESS

This exercise will strengthen the front muscles of your upper arms, which are responsible for bending your elbows and which also assist in lifting and pulling. Total time: 42 seconds.

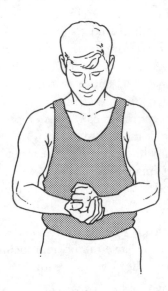

1. Stand or sit comfortably, with your arms at your sides. Bend your arms, bringing your hands to waist level (i.e., your fore-arms should be parallel to the ground).

2. Make a fist with your left hand. Cup the fist loosely in your right palm.

3. With your right hand, press upward against your left fist with as much force as you can manage. At the same time, press down against your right hand with your left fist. Hold for 2 to 3 seconds at first; gradually work up to 7 seconds of full contrac-tions.

4. Move your arms slightly higher, increasing the bend in your elbows by 10 to 15 degrees (bend them slightly more). Repeat step 3.

5. Open up your arms by moving your fists farther away from your body, so the bend in your elbow is greater than 95 de-grees. Repeat step 3.

6. Reverse the position of your hands (pushing *up* with the left and *down* with the right). Repeat all three exercises.

TRICEPS PUSH

This exercise strengthens and tones the back muscles of the upper arms, which are responsible for straightening your arms and which also assist in pushing movements. This exercise is especially good for women, who are notoriously weak in this area. Total time: 21 seconds.

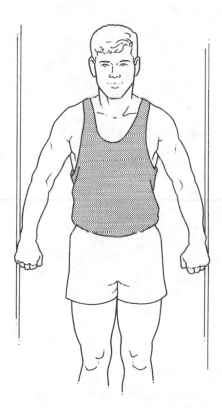

1. Stand comfortably relaxed in a doorway of average width.

2. Make fists with both hands; then, with your arms slightly bent and at hip level, push as hard as you can against the door jamb on either side. Hold for 2 to 3 seconds at first; gradually work up to 7 seconds of full contractions.

3. Bend your arms so your fists are just below shoulder level; repeat steps 1 and 2.

4. Extend your arms so your fists are just above your head. Repeat steps 1 and 2.

LAT SQUEEZE

This exercise strengthens the latissimus dorsi, the broad muscles along the side of your back, which are used to pull your arms toward your body. Total time: 14 seconds.

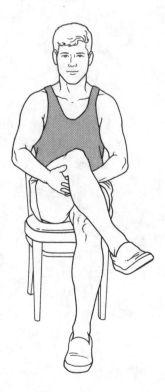

1. Sit in a firm chair with your right knee crossed over your left knee. Put both hands underneath your right knee and pull your knee strongly toward your body as hard as you can. At the same time, press forcefully downward with your knee

against your hands. Hold for 2 to 3 seconds at first; gradually work up to 7 seconds of full contractions.

2. Cross your left knee over your right and repeat the actions in step 1.

PECTORAL PUMP

This exercise strengthens your pectorals, the muscles that help you make pushing movements and that are responsible for a firm, high bustline. Total time: 21 seconds.

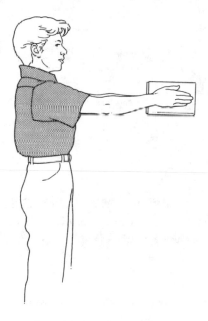

1. Stand or sit comfortably, with your arms straight out in front at shoulder level.

2. Press your hands together, then push inward with both hands, as hard as you can. (If you find it more comfortable, you may hold a book between your hands.) Hold for 2 to 3 seconds at first; gradually work up to 7 seconds of full contractions.

3. Raise your arms 10 to 15 degrees above shoulder level. Repeat steps 1 and 2.

4. Lower your arms to just below shoulder level. Repeat steps 1 and 2.

ABDOMINAL CRUNCH

This exercise strengthens your abdominal muscles, which are essential for good posture. Weak abdominals are considered by many experts to be the number-one cause of back pain. Total time: 1 to 2 minutes.

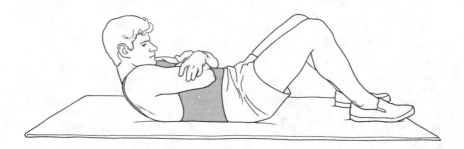

1. Lie on your back on an exercise mat or folded blanket over a firm surface. Bend your knees (your heels should be 12 to 18 inches from your buttocks) and press your lower back into the floor.

2. Crossing your arms over your chest, and tucking your chin into your chest, slowly lift your torso until your shoulder blades have cleared the floor. Hold 1 to 2 seconds; slowly return to start. Start with one to five crunches; gradually work up to fifty.

When you can easily do fifty crunches in the position indicated, you can increase the difficulty by clasping your hands behind your neck. Keep your elbows back, and be careful not to use your hands to pull your head forward.

The abdominals are truly isometric muscles—they don't go any-where. You can strengthen them all day long, in any position, in any situation. Simply "suck in your gut" (contract the abdominals) and hold for 7 seconds. Try this in the supermarket line, while waiting for the light to change, or any time you think about it. The reward will be a stronger, flatter belly.

SIDE SCRUNCH

This exercise is for the external obliques, the side abdominal muscles that enable you to turn your body from side to side or to bend to the side. Total time: 6 seconds.

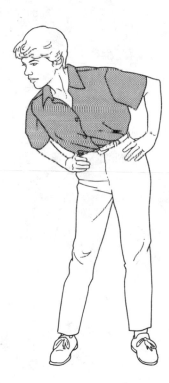

1. Stand comfortably with your hands on your hips. Pull in your abdominal muscles, hold, and slowly twist to the right side and slightly forward, as if trying to touch your hip bone with your rib cage. Hold at the extreme position for 2 to 3 seconds, at

first; gradually work up to 7 seconds of full contractions. Return to start, then proceed with step 2.

2.   Repeat step 1, twisting to the left.

GLUTEAL KICK

This exercise strengthens and tones the gluteus maximus, the large muscle that covers your buttocks, which is important in posture and walking. Total time: 14 seconds.

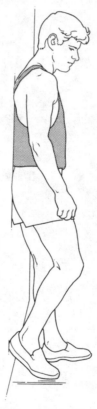

1.   Stand comfortably with your back to a wall, your feet about 4 inches from the baseboard. Raise your left heel a few inches from the floor, then press it into the wall as forcefully as you can. Hold for 2 to 3 seconds at first; gradually work up to 7 seconds of full contractions.

Note: If you have trouble keeping your balance during this exercise, you may hold onto a chair back or other piece of furniture to steady yourself.

2.   Repeat step 1, pushing your right heel against the wall.

Like your abdominals, your gluteal muscles can easily be exercised at any time and will become stronger and firmer the more frequently you contract them. For a buttocks-firming gluteal crunch, simply squeeze your buttocks together as forcefully as you can, holding the maximum contraction for a few seconds.

SIDE SWING

This exercise strengthens the abductor muscles on the outsides of your legs, which are responsible for kicking and sideways motions. Total time: 14 seconds.

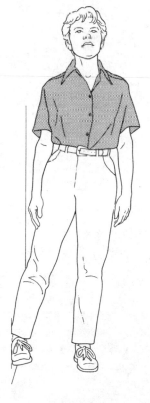

1. Stand comfortably with your right side approximately 4 inches from a wall. Swing your right leg out until it is pressed against the wall; push against the wall as forcefully as you can. Hold for 2 to 3 seconds at first; gradually work up to 7 seconds of full contractions.

2. Repeat step 1, pushing your left heel against the wall.

INNER PRESS

This exercise strengthens the adductor muscles, those often-neglected muscles along the insides of your thighs. Total time: 7 seconds.

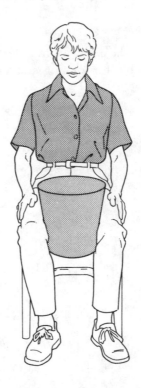

Lying on the floor or sitting, place an object like a ball, box, waste paper basket, or throw pillow between your thighs. Now squeeze your thighs together as forcefully as you can. Hold for 2 to 3 seconds at first; gradually work up to 7 seconds of full contractions. (This exercise can also be performed by squeezing the object between your knees or lower legs.)

THIGH TRIMMER

This exercise works on the quadriceps, the front part of your upper legs, important in many activities such as walking, running, lifting, or climbing stairs. Total time: 21 seconds.

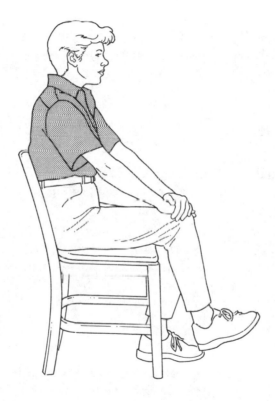

1. Sit comfortably on a chair, with your back supported and your legs bent in front of you. Place both hands slightly above the right knee and push against the knee while resisting with your thigh. Hold for 2 to 3 seconds at first; gradually work up to 7 seconds of full contractions.

2. Place both hands slightly above the left knee and repeat the actions in step 1.

3. Place your hands between your knees and push outward with your hands, while pressing inward with your knees as forcefully as you can. Hold for 2 to 3 seconds at first; gradually work up to 7 seconds of full contraction.

BONUS STRENGTHENERS

These variants of the pushup are isotonic exercises that are especially good for your back, shoulder, arm, and abdominal muscles. Start with the wall pushup and, when you have become stronger, move on to the bent-knee pushup.

WALL PUSHUP

1. Stand 1 to 2 feet from a wall with your arms straight out in front of you and your hands supporting you as you lean into the wall.

2. Slowly lower your body to the wall, then push it back out. Start with as many as you can do; build up to sixteen repetitions.

BENT-KNEE PUSHUP

1. Keeping your back straight, support yourself on your knees and outstretched palms. Your arms should be straight, your hands resting on the floor in front of you, shoulder-width apart. Your body should be at an angle to the floor.

2. Slowly lower your upper body to the ground, keeping your trunk straight and your elbows pointing straight up. Now raise yourself back to starting position. Start with as many as you can do; work up to sixteen.

The following variations of the chinup, while not practical for everyone, are especially good for your upper arms and shoulders. Both exercises require a chinning bar and are easier if you have someone to help you. (Most sporting-goods stores sell adjustable doorway chinning bars for under $10; chinning bars are also available in gyms and at most playgrounds.)

NEGATIVE CHINUP

1. Stand on a chair just under a chinning bar, holding the bar in an underhand grip (your palms facing your body). Your hands should be shoulder-width apart, and your chin should just rest on the bar.

2. Have the person assisting you move the chair away, or kick it away yourself. Hang in the same position for 3 to 5 seconds, then slowly lower your body until you are hanging by your arms or until your feet touch the ground. Repeat once or twice; work up to five.

ISOMETRIC CHINUP

Proceed as for negative chinups, above, but when your arms are bent at a 90-degree angle, hold the position for 3 to 5 seconds, or as long as you can.

PRINCETON LIFE-STYLE EXERCISES

THE Princeton Life-style Exercises are not formal exercises; rather, they are behavioral changes you can easily make in your daily routine to increase movement. In the long run these simple activities can add up to increased fitness, a higher rate of burning calories, and permanent weight loss. As you read through the next few pages you may be skeptical or feel tempted to dismiss this part of the program, thinking, "This looks too easy—how can it possibly make a difference?"

We don't blame you—life-style exercises do appear at first glance "too good to be true," but in fact it has been found that spontaneous movements and activities can use up between 100 and 900 extra calories a day! Even more encouraging, a study that compared two groups of volunteer dieters found that those who had been taught life-style exercises kept their weight off better for the long term than those who followed a programmed exercise regimen.

Irene M., a forty-one-year-old administrator, began the Princeton Plan with doubts about the value of exercise. "I used to drive everywhere," she says. "I was surprised when I found out it only took 7 minutes to walk to my office. Now I walk a lot more and climb stairs, too." She reports feeling better and having more energy since beginning the plan, and, "Of course walking helps with the weight. It made the roundness in my face disappear."

GET MOVING!

The life-style exercises we suggest are all simple and can easily become second nature, so that after a few weeks you won't even have to think about them. When you first start doing them, however, you will consciously have to keep your goals in mind and, if necessary, "psych yourself up" to exert the extra effort called for.

This is not as difficult as it may sound. What we are urging you to do is change your attitude and *think movement.* **Whenever you have a choice to make, choose the one that requires the greater amount of movement.** For example, instead of buying a long telephone cord so you don't need to get up to answer the phone, use a short cord or a wall phone. Then, every time the phone rings, you will need to work a little movement into your life. Even if it seems like a minuscule expenditure of energy, many such small choices during the day can add up to an overall big deficit in calories. In fact, a study by the Illinois Bell Telephone Company found that an extension phone saves 70 miles of walking a year—which can mean an extra 2 or 3 pounds of fat! In another dramatic example of the value of even tiny amounts of exertion, a study of secretaries who switched from manual to electric typewriters showed that most gained 1 or more pounds within a year after making the switch.

STRETCH

Stretching not only requires extra movement but also promotes flexibility and eliminates stiffness. There are many forms of stretching, including structured systems, such as hatha yoga. It is said, in fact, that this form of yoga was developed by observation of cats, who stretch at nearly every opportunity and who remain completely limber even into advanced old age.

Although we are not recommending a programmed stretching routine, here are some guidelines:

- Stretch only when your muscles are warm, to prevent injury. Just after waking in the morning is ideal; not only are your muscles warm from your blankets, the gentle activity will help to wake you up.

Another good time to stretch is after you have warmed up or completed your aerobic or strength-building program.

- Stretch as fully as you can without strain, and hold the extreme position for a few seconds. Never "bounce" when you stretch; this can cause a rebound effect that makes your muscles tighter than ever.

Below are some suggested stretches. Most suggest that you stand "comfortably"; for most people this means standing with feet approximately shoulder-width apart and knees slightly bent (*not* locked). It is not so important to follow these directions exactly as it is to stretch frequently, using as many muscles as possible, throughout the day.

- **Arm stretch.** Stand with your feet comfortably apart and your hands and arms straight overhead. Reach upward, slowly, as high as possible with one hand, as if you were trying to touch the ceiling. Hold at the extreme position for a few seconds, then reach slowly with the other hand. Repeat several times with each hand.

- **Side stretch.** Stand with your feet comfortably apart and your right hand on your waist, your left arm overhead. Now gently bend to the right side until you feel a stretching on your left side. Hold for a few seconds, then switch the positions of your hands and bend to the other side. Repeat several times on each side.

- **Leg stretch.** Stand comfortably with your arms relaxed. Keeping your back straight, shift your weight to your left leg and raise your right knee toward your chest, pulling it as high as possible with your hands. Hold for 1 or 2 seconds, then extend the leg, as if you were kicking a football. Lower the leg, then shift your weight to your right foot and repeat both actions with your left knee. Repeat two or three times on each side.

  In the same position, lean slightly forward, lift your right leg backward, with knee bent, as far as you can. Imagine that you are trying to touch the back of your head with your heel. Hold for a second or two, then lower the leg and repeat with your left leg. Repeat two or three times on each side.

- **Twist.** Stand comfortably with your arms outstretched to the front at shoulder level. Imagine that you are holding a broomstick in your hands. Keeping your arms outstretched and a couple of inches apart, twist your entire trunk to the right, your arms moving with it. (Your right arm will be stretched to the right side, your left arm crossed to the right over your trunk.) Swing back to center and then to the left. Repeat rhythmically.

DON'T SAVE YOURSELF EXTRA STEPS

A young woman we know, who is constantly trying to watch her weight, prides herself on her efficiency. Instead of taking items from downstairs upstairs whenever needed, she stores them at the bottom of the stairs until she has several things to take upstairs at once. While this may be commendable in terms of efficiency, it is counterproductive to her desired weight loss. Each trip upstairs would take only a few seconds but would help burn calories and build muscle in her legs.

You may not live in a home with stairs, but there are undoubtedly many ways in which you can add just a little movement to your day. For example, do you often find yourself asking a family member to bring you something (a glass of soda, the newspaper)? Get out of your chair and get it yourself. Even better, volunteer to bring things to others in the household.

There are many other ways you can make sure that extra steps are built into your day. For example, install the washing machine in the basement instead of the kitchen; park your car or get off the bus a little further from your office than normal; walk a memo to your colleague instead of sending it through interoffice mail; whenever possible, use stairs instead of elevators or escalators, even if only for one flight.

FORGET MODERN CONVENIENCES

It is true that most modern appliances are intended to save labor as well as time, and certainly in today's busy world few of us have time to return to doing things by hand on a regular basis. Still, try to make time, if only occasionally, for doing by hand at least some of the tasks you now perform by machine:

- Rake leaves instead of using a leaf blower. Besides working up a good sweat, this activity can be pleasing and a source of fun for the whole family.

- Use a hand mower rather than an electric mower.

- Hang clothes on the line instead of using the drier (this is especially good in sunny weather—clothes hung outside to dry acquire a fresh, sun-filled scent).

- Prepare some food dishes by hand rather than using a blender, food processor, or electric beater.

- "Just say no" to TV and do something more active, even if it's merely taking a leisurely walk or playing a game with friends.

PRACTICE "CREATIVE FIDGETING"

Have you ever known a skinny person who claims that "nervous energy" keeps his or her weight down? This is more than an old wives' tale. Some people just naturally move more than others—you see them tapping their fingers or swinging their legs. While such habits can be annoying, and we don't recommend them, spontaneous movement all through the day can burn a large number of calories. If you have been sedentary for many years you may find it difficult to be truly "spontaneous" in your movements, but the more you become accustomed to movement, the easier it will get. Stretch several times a day. Stand rather than sit; stoop, squat, reach, move your body as many ways as you can whenever you think of it.

Remember, *any* movement is better than none. Sitting uses more energy than lying down; standing uses more energy than sitting; and walking uses more energy than standing. See the following table for calories expended for various activities.

THE COMPLETE PRINCETON
EXERCISE/EATING PLAN

You have learned about all the parts of the complete Princeton Plan: the low/high-calorie alternating diet and the three-part exercise pro-

---

CALORIES BURNED PER HOUR
(By Healthy 150-Pound Adult)

Lying down	80–100
Sitting	85–105
Standing	100–120
Walking slowly	210–230
Walking quickly	315–345
Cleaning house	125–310
Shopping	125–310
Gardening	315–480
Shoveling snow	480–625

---

gram. Now you are ready to combine healthful eating and exercise for the greatest possible increase in thermogenesis and weight loss.

Just as the *types* of food and exercise are keys to the success of the Princeton Plan, so is the relative *timing* of each part in relation to the others. Although there are a number of myths about food and athletic performance, one of the most widespread is that a precompetition meal is important. In fact, the opposite is the case. The truth, as physiologists have discovered, is that the most important meal for today's activities is the one you ate *yesterday*. In other words, the fuel your muscles "burn" for energy comes from the previous day's intake. The two primary fuels are, as we explained earlier, glycogen, a form of starch stored in muscles and the liver, and fat. Your body has a virtually unlimited ability to store fat, but the amount of sugar it can keep on hand is strictly limited, and taking advantage of this fact can actually maximize the amount of fat burned.

Thus, food eaten on the high-carbohydrate day increases your body's stores of glycogen. These stores are then used the next day when you do your muscle-building exercises, which are anaerobic and must be fueled entirely by stored glycogen. The following day, your glycogen stores are lower (after the low-carbohydrate day), making it easier for you to burn fat during your aerobic routine.

Remember that every facet of the complete Princeton Plan is designed to maximize weight loss. Alternating high- and low-calorie days is essential to prevent metabolic slowdown and the plateau effect, while the three parts of the exercise program will speed weight loss and ensure that it lasts.

THE COMPLETE PRINCETON EXERCISE/EATING PLAN

Day One

    Diet: low-carbohydrate, low-calorie

    Exercise:
- warmup before strength-building exercise
- strength-building exercise, preferably before largest meal of the day
- some aerobics (remember that for weight loss, five to six days of aerobics produces best results)
- life-style exercises all day long

Day Two

    Diet: high-carbohydrate, high-calorie

    Exercise:
- warmup before aerobic exercise
- aerobic exercise before largest meal of the day
- life-style exercises all day long

Simply continue to alternate the plans offered in Day One and Day Two. For anyone who wants to go farther, and further increase thermogenesis, or use the Princeton Plan principles to improve athletic performance, the next section offers a number of optional strategies for increasing the effectiveness of the basic program.

PART IV

PUTTING IT
ALL TOGETHER

STICKING WITH IT

BECAUSE we have worked with dieters for many years, we realize that you may be tempted, especially if you have tried unsuccessfully to lose weight in the past, to think of the Princeton Plan as just another diet. We hope you don't, because that attitude toward dieting has helped to keep you overweight. The only way to make long term changes in your life is to change your attitude toward food and dieting. And the best way to change your attitude is to change your behavior.

This may sound contradictory, but behavioral psychologists have proven that it is true: *Behavior* changes *precede* attitude changes. This principle is, in fact, one of the foundations of the therapy known as **behavior modification**. Behavior modification makes use of a number of strategies, such as self-monitoring, or recording your own behavior (for example, noting exactly when, where, and what you eat); stimulus control, which attempts to reduce or eliminate the stimuli that lead to undesirable activity (for example, keeping fattening foods out of sight); and behavior change, in which you consciously alter a previous habitual behavior (for example, chewing each bite thoroughly, rather than wolfing down your food).

The purpose of each of these techniques is to make it easier for you to form new, desirable habits: eating appropriate quantities of whole-

some and nutrient-rich foods, and exercising on a regular basis. You
have probably heard some of these strategies before; many of them are
well known because they have been proven, over time, to work. We
aren't asking you to adopt all the suggestions that follow but rather to
pick the ones you think might work for you and give them a try.

KEEP A RECORD

In classical behavior-modification therapy, keeping a record, or self-
monitoring, is one of the most important and useful tools, because it
can make you *consciously* aware of your behavior and what triggers it.
It can also serve to reinforce and perpetuate new, desirable habits.

An example of the first application is to keep a food diary. If you
have not yet started the Princeton Eating Plan, you may find it useful
to begin your eating diary now. In it, write down everything you ate
during the day, where and when you ate it, and what the circumstances
were (it was lunchtime, you were angry at your boss, etc.). After a few
days, review the diary in the light of the things you have learned about
the Princeton Eating Plan. For example, although your overall calorie
consumption may not be high, note how many foods that you eat do
not contribute to or even work against thermogenesis. Also notice
where you eat and the circumstances; you may discover patterns that
can help you to avoid situations that may tempt you to overeat.

Continue to keep your eating diary after you begin the Eating Plan;
simply recording your intake will help you become more familiar with
how the plan works and will also help you monitor the circumstances
surrounding any "slips" you may make. Irene M., one of our most
successful clients, credits her food diary with helping to change long-
standing eating habits: "It helped me learn the food exchanges," she
explains, "and for the first time I became aware it's *food* I'm eating, not
just calories."

Keeping a record is perhaps even more important for the Princeton
Exercise Plan and serves two purposes: keeping track of the amount
of exercise you have done; and, by showing steady progress, serving
as an incentive to keep you going.

You will need to keep separate records for the two formal parts of
the exercise program, but these needn't be elaborate. For the strength-

building exercises, simply note how many of each exercise you did during each session and how many seconds you held that position. A sample chart, filled out for three weeks, can be found on page 202. A blank chart for your own use can be found on pages 203–205.

For your aerobic program, you also need just a simple record, such as the one shown on pages 206–209. When you first begin, simply note how much time you spent on the activity. (For example: "Monday—walked 10 minutes.") As you become more aerobically fit, your exercise record will reflect your increased endurance, providing a real reinforcement on those days when you just don't feel like exercising.

Once you have reached the maintenance level of aerobic exercise, record-keeping can help you avoid becoming bored. If your activity is walking, jogging, bicycling, or swimming, you may want to keep a record of the distances you have logged. Some walkers and joggers keep cumulative totals and plot them on a chart or graph. You can even mark your progress on a map—it can give you quite a sense of accomplishment to "walk" the miles from, say, Minneapolis to Phoenix.

Keeping records can also keep you from getting discouraged if you feel you aren't improving. Looking back over the record provides positive proof of how much progress you have made so far.

A final way to use record-keeping is to keep track of weight and/or inches lost. Plotted on a graph, the steady decline can provide a vivid representation of your continued success on the Princeton Plan.

GET A BUDDY

If at all possible, try to find someone else to join you on one or both parts of the Princeton Plan. This strategy can help in several ways, the most obvious being that "misery loves company." Not that you will be miserable on the Plan—quite the opposite. But because any diet is by nature restrictive, it can help to have someone to commiserate with and talk to when you feel a "slip" coming on.

Having an exercise buddy is an excellent way of ensuring that you will do your exercises regularly. If you make a firm date to work out with someone, you will be less likely to give in to the temptation to "skip it just this once," because you won't want to let your buddy down. Or, as one Princeton dieter, who takes late-night walks with a

Exercise	Start/ Goal	Position	Week 1			Week 2			Week 3		
Biceps Press	3 Sec/ 7 Sec Ea. Side	Straight	3	3	3	4	4	5	5	5	5
		Up	3	3	3	4	4	5	5	5	5
		Down	3	3	3	4	4	5	5	5	5
Triceps Push	3 Sec/ 7 Sec	Hip	3	3	3	4	4	5	5	5	5
		Shoulder	3	3	3	4	4	5	5	5	5
		Head	3	3	3	4	4	5	5	5	5
Lat Squeeze	3 Sec/ 7 Sec Ea. Side		3	3	3	4	4	5	5	5	5
Pectoral Pump	3 Sec/ 7 Sec	Shoulder	3	3	3	4	4	5	5	5	5
		Up	3	3	3	4	4	5	5	5	5
		Down	3	3	3	4	4	5	5	5	5
Adominal Crunch	1–5x/ 50x		1	1	1	2	2	2	3	3	4
Side Scrunch	2–3 Sec/ 7 Sec										
Gluteal Kick	3 Sec/ 7 Sec Ea. Side		3	3	3	4	4	5	5	5	5
Side Swing	3 Sec/ 7 Sec Ea. Side		3	3	3	4	4	5	5	5	5
Inner Press	3 Sec/ 7 Sec		3	3	3	4	4	5	5	5	5
Thigh Trimmer	3 Sec/ 7 Sec	Right	3	3	3	4	4	5	5	5	5
		Left	3	3	3	4	4	5	5	5	5
		Between	3	3	3	4	4	5	5	5	5
*Pushup	1x/16x		1	1	1	2	1	2	2	2	3
*Chinup	1x/5x		1	1	1	1	1	1	1	1	2

Exercise	Start/ Goal	Position	Week 1		Week 2		Week 3	
Biceps Press	3 Sec/ 7 Sec Ea. Side	Straight						
		Up						
		Down						
Triceps Push	3 Sec/ 7 Sec	Hip						
		Shoulder						
		Head						
Lat Squeeze	3 Sec/ 7 Sec Ea. Side							
Pectoral Pump	3 Sec/ 7 Sec	Shoulder						
		Up						
		Down						
Abdominal Crunch	1–5x/ 50x							
Side Scrunch	2–3 Sec/ 7 Sec							
Gluteal Kick	3 Sec/ 7 Sec Ea. Side							
Side Swing	3 Sec/ 7 Sec Ea. Side							
Inner Press	3 Sec/ 7 Sec							
Thigh Trimmer	3 Sec/ 7 Sec	Right						
		Left						
		Between						
*Pushup	1x/16x							
*Chinup	1x/5x							

Week 4	Week 5	Week 6	Week 7	Week 8	Week 9	Week 10

Week 11	Week 12	Week 13	Week 14	Week 15	Week 16	Week 17

Week	Day	Progress	Comment
1	1	Walk 5 min	feel good
	2	Walk 5 min	so far so good
	3	Walk 5 min	
	4	Walk 5 min	feel tired
	5		no time
2	1	Walk 5 min	good—ready for more
	2	Walk 6 min	as easy as 5!
	3	Walk 6 min	good
	4	Walk 5 min	tired today
	5	Walk 7 min	feel very strong!
3	1	Walk 7 min	legs look trimmer
	2	Walk 7 min	
	3	Walk 5 min	ankles sore—stopped early
	4		
	5		
4	1		
	2		
	3		
	4		
	5		
5	1		
	2		
	3		
	4		
	5		

Week	Day	Progress	Comment
1	1		
	2		
	3		
	4		
	5		
2	1		
	2		
	3		
	4		
	5		
3	1		
	2		
	3		
	4		
	5		
4	1		
	2		
	3		
	4		
	5		
5	1		
	2		
	3		
	4		
	5		

Week	Day	Progress	Comment
6	1		
	2		
	3		
	4		
	5		
7	1		
	2		
	3		
	4		
	5		
8	1		
	2		
	3		
	4		
	5		
9	1		
	2		
	3		
	4		
	5		
10	1		
	2		
	3		
	4		
	5		

Week	Day	Progress	Comment
11	1		
	2		
	3		
	4		
	5		
12	1		
	2		
	3		
	4		
	5		
13	1		
	2		
	3		
	4		
	5		
14	1		
	2		
	3		
	4		
	5		
15	1		
	2		
	3		
	4		
	5		

partner, puts it, "No matter how exhausted I am, I don't make a telephone call to cancel. If she can do it, I can do it."

FOLLOW A REGULAR SCHEDULE

On any diet or exercise regimen, it is important to follow a regular schedule, both to make sure that you observe all parts of the program and because your body likes regularity—it gets used to eating at the same time and exercising at the same time. Following a schedule is even more important on the Princeton Plan, because the diet and exercise plans increase thermogenesis most effectively when followed exactly as we have described them.

When planning your own schedule, adapt the Princeton guidelines as much as possible to your own preferences and life-style. But remember that aerobic exercise works best to stimulate thermogenesis when performed before the largest meal of the day. Furthermore, evidence indicates that working out in the daytime elevates your metabolism for a longer period than nighttime exercise. Remember, too, that calories eaten late at night are stored more efficiently as fat; try to eat dinner by 7:00 P.M.

MAKE IT PLEASANT

This too seems obvious, but many people have such a negative attitude toward diet and exercise that they unconsciously go out of their way to make the experience less pleasant than it might be.

When you prepare your meals, for example, don't think of them as "just diet food"; rather, think of them as tasty and healthful meals. Set good dishes and flatware on place mats or a nice tablecloth. Eat by candlelight, if you like. Regard your meals as special occasions on which you are doing something nice for yourself.

By the same token, make your exercise routine as pleasant as possible. When you are doing the strength-building exercises, turn on your favorite music. Make sure that the room is comfortably cool (turn on the fan or air conditioner). Invest in a portable radio or tape player with earphones for your walking program, and listen to your favorite music while you exercise. Or get a tape of a book that you have been meaning to read, and improve your mind while you improve the condition of your heart, lungs, and circulatory system.

THINK POSITIVELY

This approach is related to the preceding one; you might think of it as emphasizing willpower over "won't" power. As described by nutrition writer Barbara Gibbons, "won't power" is a negative mind-set toward dieting in which you focus on the things you are giving up rather than the benefits you are receiving.

It's easy to avoid obsessing on the negative—simply learn to frame your thoughts about the Princeton Plan in a positive way. Instead of saying, "I can't have takeout hamburgers anymore," think, "I'm going to have a delicious homemade burger with a whole-wheat roll and lots of veggies."

Instead of mourning gooey, fatty, sugary desserts (which always made you feel guilty anyway), celebrate the fact that on the Princeton Plan you are allowed several generous helpings a day of fresh fruits.

Whenever you find yourself slipping into negative attitudes, turn the thought around and focus instead on the positive, healthful aspects of your plan.

BE PREPARED

Be prepared for the fact that you may have setbacks, in either or both parts of the program, and don't let them upset you. For example, if you fall off the diet occasionally and eat some forbidden foods, simply accept that you are human, and return to the diet where you left it. Remember that supermarkets, television, and print ads are all working against you, urging you to eat unhealthful foods that are designed to make you fat. It is difficult to avoid temptation under these circumstances. And don't worry—the longer you remain on the Princeton Eating Plan, the easier it will be to stay on it, because the foods you formerly ate will no longer taste as good to you as they once did.

Be prepared also for the possibility that a family member or a friend may try to sabotage your efforts. Psychologists know that very often when someone in a family or friendship circle begins making changes in behavior, whether these changes are for the better or the worse, it can upset the dynamics of the circle. In consequence, other members of the group may subconsciously try to sabotage the new behavior. For example, members of your family might complain, "We're having rice and beans again? Yuck!" You may have to spend extra time preparing separate dishes for your family, but it will be worth it. Likewise, friends or family may comment that you don't "need" to lose weight or that you aren't fun any more. Simply ignore them, and continue with your Plan.

Be prepared as well for the possibility that you will not readily lose weight on the basic plan presented in previous chapters. This is more likely the more overweight you are or the more often you have unsuccessfully dieted in the past. If you haven't lost any weight by the end of the third week on the Plan, then you may need to go on a lower-calorie diet. Turn to Appendix A for complete instructions on how to plan menus for diets within a wide calorie range.

On the other hand, you may lose weight yet find yourself constantly hungry. If this is the case, then you probably need to *increase* your basic calorie allowance. Appendix A can help you plan your new menus. Remember, you should never feel excessively hungry on this diet! Some hunger near mealtimes is normal and healthy.

It is important to learn the difference between hunger and appetite, by the way. Hunger is a *physical* reaction, while appetite is *emotional*. Genuine hunger is usually accompanied by stomach pangs or growling, which can be temporarily relieved by drinking a glass of water or tightening your belt. Appetite is an emotional longing for a particular food or more of a given food and is often perpetuated by the sight, smell, or taste of the food itself. For this reason, try to avoid situations and places that might stimulate your appetite: Stay out of bakeries, do not put serving dishes on the table, and, whenever possible, leave the table promptly when you have finished eating.

BE REALISTIC

As fallible humans, we are all prey to bouts of wishful thinking; going on a diet—and especially one that is successful—often triggers fantasies about how wonderful life will be once one's goal weight is reached. It is true that weight loss can make a big difference in the quality of your life; most successful Princeton dieters report improved energy and stamina and a general feeling of health and well-being. But except for giving you the energy to make other positive changes, losing weight will *not* affect other parts of your life that are less than satisfactory: It will not change the shape of your nose, turn you into a movie star, or produce a winning lottery ticket.

To avoid unrealistic expectations, it may help to remind yourself consciously *why* you are following the Princeton Plan, especially if you begin to feel anxious or depressed. Improved appearance, health, and well-being are realistic goals. Remember, too, that you are making these positive changes for yourself and nobody else. If you also happen to win the lottery, that is a bonus, but it has nothing to do with the Princeton Plan.

You can also help to reduce your anxieties by changing the way you dress, cultivating a slimmer appearance as you gradually shed pounds. For both men and women, solid colors are best, avoid plaids, large prints, and horizontal stripes. Women can camouflage figure faults with scarves and loose tops, but beware of clothes that are too loose, which can look sloppy and hide the progress you have made. The other extreme—buying a whole new wardrobe in size 6—can also be self-defeating, presenting a goal that may be far away or unrealistic for you. A better strategy is to add new items to your wardrobe gradually. Look for clothing with elasticized waists that will continue to fit as you grow thinner.

REWARD YOURSELF

Behavioral scientists know that one of the best ways to reinforce positive behavior is to offer rewards—and you can do this yourself. Promise yourself a special treat (but not food!) when you have lost a certain amount of weight. Schedule these rewards on a regular basis. You can also reward yourself as you become more fit as a result of the exercise portion of the Plan. For example, buy a new warmup suit once you have reached 20 minutes of exercise. Not only can this make you feel "athletic," its sleek look will give you tangible proof that you are getting thinner.

EDUCATE YOURSELF

We hope that what you have read so far in this book has made you more interested in nutrition and exercise. If so, then finding out more will help make it easier for you to stick to all parts of the Plan. Check out some library books on nutrition and exercise, or subscribe to a health-oriented magazine. A reading list is included in Appendix D to get you started.

MAKE IT EASY ON YOURSELF

The following tips can all make your new eating and exercise plans easier to follow. Look them over—and try them.

- **When preparing meals, cook ahead**, then freeze "Princeton-sized" portions to be used at future meals. This is not only a time saver but also can help you continue to follow the diet when you just aren't in the mood to prepare a meal.

- Eat slowly. Studies show that a majority of overweight people eat more quickly than leaner folks. Eating fast is an invitation to overeating, because it takes approximately 20 minutes for your brain to get the message that you are "full." Strategies for slowing down your eating pace include taking small bites; chewing your food thoroughly; and putting your fork down between bites. If you know how to eat with chopsticks, use them at any meal where it is appropriate; this will also help slow down your eating pace.

- **Eat dinner before 7:00 P.M.** This will help ensure that you aren't digesting your food when you sleep, which can encourage the storage of extra fat.

- **Carry a baggie of "free" veggies around** with you all day so you will be prepared when you want a snack.

- **Focus on your progress,** not your shortcomings. Take note of the clothes that are becoming looser and the extra amount of energy and stamina you have, rather than how far you still have to go.

- **When you eat, don't do anything else.** Eating while watching television or talking on the phone can sabotage the best-intended plans. When we're distracted, it's very easy to lose track of how much we are eating or fail to notice when our body signals that we have had enough. Always eat in the same place (e.g., dining room, kitchen table). Don't eat standing up. And never eat anything directly out of the package.

- **Never go food shopping when you are hungry!** It's too easy to fall prey to those appetizing displays of unhealthful junk foods. Don't buy foods on impulse; rather, use a shopping list. Try to do all of your shopping for the week at once, to avoid further temptations in the supermarket.

- **Make a family activity out of planning meals.** This tip was contributed by one of our clients, who sits down with her husband and children to plan weekly menus. "The kids have gotten interested in helping me lose weight," she reports, "and I feel they're learning good nutrition."

- **Get rid of unhealthful foods** and snacks, or, if your family insists on keeping them around, make sure they are well hidden.

- **If you need to eat, eat.** One of our clients, who used to stuff herself with cheese and crackers after work, jokes that she now "binges on carrots and lettuce." "When I get off work I'm hungry and have no patience to wait for dinner," she says. So she allows herself to eat a big bowl of raw veggies, which takes the edge off her hunger and gets her through to dinner.

- **Make a "snack bag."** This is another tip from one of our successful dieters, who prepares a plastic bag containing her daily snacks and some free veggies before she goes to work in the morning.

- **Set realistic goals.** You didn't gain your excess weight in a week, and you're not going to lose it in a week. A reasonable amount of weight loss is 1 to 3 pounds per week. Likewise, don't overdo your exercise. Slow and steady wins the race.

- **Drink plenty of water.** Most Americans do not drink enough water, and exercise will increase your need for this vital fluid. Drinking up to eight glasses of pure spring water a day will help you avoid feelings of hunger and may increase your stamina and improve your complexion as well.

- **Get a hobby.** This may seem like a strange suggestion, but taking up an activity that keeps your hands and mind busy can help you avoid the temptation to snack in the evenings. Needle-work, stamp collecting, or model building can help keep you slim.

- **If you find the Princeton-sized portions depressingly small, serve them on a salad plate** instead of a dinner plate. This increases the apparent size of the portion and can help prevent any feelings of deprivation.

MAKING THE PRINCETON PLAN A PART OF YOUR LIFE

MAINTENANCE

STUDIES show that the time when dieters are most likely to fail is when they get to within a few pounds of their weight-loss goal or have reached it. In most cases, the reason for this seeming self-sabotage is a failure to adopt healthy eating habits permanently. A man we know who lost 90 pounds on a conventional diet regained almost 40 within a few weeks of reaching maintenance. "I couldn't handle all the freedom," he admitted. "It was around Thanksgiving time and I saw all that food and I just went nuts."

In other words, our friend reverted to the same eating habits that had made him fat in the first place, and it is this tendency that is one of the major problems with traditional diets: Once the weight is lost, dieters go back to their former way of eating. *No diet,* including the Princeton Plan, can work for the long term unless it results in a *permanent* change in eating behavior. We have designed the Princeton Plan so that you can easily follow its basic principles for a lifetime.

With that understanding, you will probably find maintenance easier on the Princeton Plan than on any other regimen you have tried.

For one thing, our alternation of low- and high-calorie days prevents the metabolic slowdown that usually accompanies dieting, so you will not quickly start to regain weight in a rebound effect as you increase your caloric intake. Secondly, because the Princeton Plan provides complete nutrition, you should not feel undue cravings to begin eating the unhealthful foods you have been "deprived" of.

Maintenance on the Princeton Plan consists of continuing to eat healthful whole foods but in greater amounts and in a less structured way. Although you needn't follow the exchange allowances as strictly as you did on the weight-loss plan, continue to alternate low-calorie, low-carbohydrate days with high-calorie, high-carbohydrate days. When you get within 5 pounds of your goal weight, you may begin to increase the exchanges that you eat each day or to increase portions. You may also add small amounts of meat on the high-carbohydrate days or enjoy an occasional glass of wine with dinner. (Do not have more than one drink per day, however. Alcoholic beverages not only contain empty calories, they can affect your judgment and cause you to revert to unhealthful eating habits.)

If you begin to regain lost pounds, return to the regimen you followed to lose weight steadily. You will need to experiment to discover your new "core" calorie count (the number of calories you alternate around), but as long as you continue to eat the Princeton way, you will probably find you can eat noticeably more than you did before beginning the Plan, without gaining weight.

Continue to take the recommended supplements and to follow the three-part exercise program. Weigh yourself at least once a week, and if you gain 5 pounds, return to the basic Princeton Plan for a few days or weeks.

Although by now your healthy new way of eating and exercising should be a part of your life, even beneficial habits can sometimes become tedious. If you find yourself becoming "stale," now may be the time to put more variety into your exercise program: Begin to jog or swim instead of walk; join an aerobics class; enroll in a weight-training program at a local gym.

THE PRINCETON PLAN AND YOUR FAMILY

Unlike traditional and "crash" diets, the Princeton Plan can be followed by the whole family; simply give your spouse and children larger portions (but bear in mind that children under four should not eat a diet restricted in fat).

If you and your family have been eating the typical American diet for many years, you may find that your loved ones balk at eating lower-fat, low-salt foods made with whole ingredients. This may be especially true of teenagers. If so, introduce them to the Princeton Plan gradually: Slowly eliminate excess salt and saturated and processed fats; introduce whole-food ingredients a little at a time until everyone has a chance to get used to them. Many people, for example, dislike whole-wheat pasta the first time they try it, so make pasta dishes with ¼ whole-grain pasta and ¾ white-flour pasta (whole-grain pastas take longer to cook than those made of white flour, so add them to the boiling water at different times). Gradually increase the proportion of whole-grain pasta to white.

As much as possible, stick to favorite family dishes, so this new way of eating won't seem so strange. For example, if your family loves red meat, continue to serve it, but not as often or in as great quantities. Choose leaner cuts and prepare them in healthier ways. For example, grill rather than fry hamburgers; cook roasts on a rack so the fat can drip off; remove all visible fat from pork, beef, or lamb cuts before cooking. Use meat as a condiment, in salads and stir-fry dishes.

In one large family we know, the six children refused at first to eat plain steamed vegetables. Their mother, whose doctor had advised her to lose weight, tried sprinkling a small amount of grated cheese on the veggies and gradually won over her toughest critics. Eventually she was able to cut back and then eliminate the cheese for all but the youngest child.

Fran C., another busy mother, jokes that converting her family to the Princeton Plan was no problem because "they complain no matter what I serve." On a more serious note, she explains that cooking the Princeton way has forced her to be more creative in the kitchen, resulting in many new dishes that everyone in the family likes. "They eat what I do," she says, "except I serve them meat every night."

To help your family eat as healthfully as possible between meals (and to reduce temptation for yourself), keep a supply of healthful snacks on hand at all times: fresh fruit, vegetable sticks, and sunflower and pumpkin seeds.

ADAPTING FAMILY RECIPES

When adapting family recipes to the Princeton Plan, keep three basic guidelines in mind. First, replace refined foods with whole ones. (For example, in a family lasagna recipe, substitute whole-wheat noodles for white noodles.) Second, eliminate as much fat as possible (use PAM instead of greasing the lasagna pan; sauté the onions and other sauce ingredients in PAM). Third, cut down on (or make substitutions for) calorie-dense foods. Instead of ricotta cheese, try low-fat cottage cheese, or combine the two cheeses in equal parts. Use only enough sausage for flavoring, or try a vegetarian lasagna, using PAM-sautéed zucchini or eggplant. Reduce the amount of Parmesan cheese you sprinkle on, adding only enough for flavoring.

EATING OUT

We will not pretend that it is always easy to follow the Princeton Plan when eating out, because in many cases it isn't. Still, as one of our clients discovered to her delight, "You don't have to turn into a hermit to lose weight." The important thing is to be aware that, sadly, most restaurants still offer typical selections from the standard American diet, full of excess salt and sugar, as well as rich sauces, gravies, and dressings made from processed oils and saturated fats.

The good news is that with a little planning and effort it is possible to follow Princeton guidelines when dining out. And even better news is that a growing number of restaurants are willing to modify food preparation in response to customers' requests. Even fast-food chains are beginning to get into the act, offering "lighter" versions of some of their popular meals, and even packaged salads. We recommend that you eat in those places only as a last resort, however, because their foods are usually oversalted and contain preservatives.

When eating at a sit-down restaurant, you must be assertive and ask

for what you want. If the management refuses to cooperate, go elsewhere; but we think you will find, as we have, that more and more
restaurants are catering to a health-conscious clientele. Although you
may not be able to find exactly what you want, you can almost always
find something that fits the healthful guidelines of the way you eat now.
And remember that unless you are eating at a health-food restaurant
that specializes in dishes made from complex carbohydrates, you will
probably find it easier to eat out on your low-calorie, low-carbohydrate
days than on your high-carbohydrate days.

Whenever you eat out, observe the following guidelines:

- **Be assertive.** Don't be afraid to ask your waiter how food is
prepared or to request that it be modified. For example, ask that
your fish be broiled without butter and that vegetables be
served plain. Ask for extra lemon, if you like, to replace butter
or fatty sauces. Ask that your food be prepared without extra
salt or MSG (monosodium glutamate), which is also high in
sodium. Many restaurants, even Chinese ones, are becoming
accustomed to customers' requests to cut back on salt.

  Instead of mayonnaise, ask for mustard only on sandwiches,
and ask for yogurt or cottage cheese to top your baked potato.
If they are not available, lemon juice is an acceptable moistener.

- **Emphasize wholesome foods.** Always have a salad with your
meal, but ask that it be served with olive oil and vinegar on the
side (olive oil contains healthful monounsaturated fats). If you
order a tuna salad, ask that it be served without mayonnaise,
because commercial mayonnaise may contain partially hydrogenated oils. When given a choice of vegetables, opt for
those that are steamed or raw. Many restaurants offer a choice
between brown and processed (white) rice; select the whole
grain. Ask for whole-wheat rolls, if possible, and request fresh
fruit for dessert.

  If the restaurant has a salad bar, load up on raw vegetables,
sunflower seeds, and beans. But beware of salad-bar pastas,
pâtés, and anything in a marinade. These are generally very
high in processed fat and salt.

- **Avoid alcohol,** or limit yourself to one alcoholic drink at the
most. Instead, ask for mineral water with a twist of lime, or fruit
or vegetable juice.

- **Don't overdo.** Because restaurant portions are often large, it is easy to overeat without realizing it. To avoid this temptation, employ any of the following strategies: Split an entree with another person; order an appetizer instead of an entree; ask for a child's portion; or take half the meal home in a doggie bag.

Eating on the Princeton Plan does not mean that you have to forego your favorite ethnic delights; in fact, some ethnic cuisines, because they are based on complex carbohydrates, are among the most healthful choices on any menu. The following guidelines for selecting healthful foods in ethnic restaurants are adapted from *Nutrition Action,* a publication of the Center for Science in the Public Interest:

Cajun. Fish (without butter), shrimp creole, and jambalaya are all low-fat, tasty winners. But avoid *estouffades,* deep-fried crawfish or shrimp, and "dirty" rice, which is loaded with saturated fat.

Chinese. The most healthful choices are stir-fried dishes that combine small amounts of seafood, poultry, or meat with fresh vegetables. Avoid dishes made with heavy sauces and such greasy entrees as Peking duck, egg foo yong, crispy fish, chicken, or shrimp, and fried dim sum.

French. Most dishes poached or cooked in wine sauce fit in with the Princeton guidelines. Avoid sweetbreads, pig's feet, sausage, liver and pâté, quiches, and anything in a cream sauce.

Indian. Most Indian dishes are relatively low in fat and high in complex carbohydrates. Especially good are dals, vegetable curries, biryani and pilaf, tandoori chicken and fish, nan, and chapati. Avoid dishes made with ghee (clarified butter) or coconut milk (ask your waiter if you are not sure of a dish's ingredients) and fried breads such as poori and paratha.

Italian. As with French food, choose dishes made with tomato or wine sauces, while avoiding those with cream sauces and heavy additions of cheese. Especially healthful are pasta primavera or marinara, pasta with red clam sauce, and minestrone. Foods to watch out for include veal or chicken parmigiana, pesto sauce, and lasagne.

Japanese. Much Japanese food is highly salted, but it is one of the lowest-fat cuisines available. Choose fish or chicken teriyaki, most soups, *yakimono* (broiled) fish and chicken. Avoid batter-fried foods such as fish and vegetable tempura, tonkatsu (pork), torikatsu (chicken), and katsudon (pork and egg). Although sushi and sashimi are low in fat and high in omega-3 oils, most experts now advise against eating raw fish because of the dangers of contamination by pollutants or parasites.

Mexican. Many Mexican (and Tex-Mex) dishes can be very healthful, because they are high in complex carbohydrates and the chiles contain capsaicin, a thermogenic agent. Good choices are seviche (marinated seafood) and bean, seafood, or chicken burritos or enchiladas without extra cheese. Stay away from anything prepared with lard, such as refried beans (again, ask your waiter), and dishes that are fried or stuffed with cheese, like chimichangas, tostadas, and cheese enchiladas.

Middle eastern/Greek. Another good choice, high in complex carbohydrates and generally low in fat. Especially good are meat and vegetable shish kabobs, couscous, pilafs, and tabbuli. Avoid deep-fried foods like falafel, kibbeh (lamb and butter), and spinach pie (spanokopita).

HOW TO HANDLE PARTIES AND HOLIDAYS

Probably the most difficult obstacle for anyone trying to eat a healthful diet is the temptations offered during parties and holiday times. Not only are we subjected to a bewildering array of fattening foods and desserts; there is enormous social pressure to consume more than a moderate amount of such offerings. The result is usually weight gain and guilt.

To survive dinners and cocktail parties, it may help to follow these guidelines: Before you attend a party, especially a dinner party, tell your host or hostess that you are on a diet to improve your health, and explain what foods you are eating and how they are prepared. Offer to bring your own meal so she or he doesn't need to go to extra trouble. Or offer to bring a side dish—perhaps steamed vegetables and rice—that you can eat as your main dish and other guests can share.

If the hostess is serving only snacks, offer to bring a tray of crudités—sliced raw vegetables—and a low-fat dip, perhaps yogurt and herbs, so you will have an alternative to greasy chips and slabs of cheese and pâté.

Before leaving home, have a good-size snack, such as fruit and sunflower seeds, so you won't get hungry when faced with the array of fattening "treats." Resist pressure to "just taste" or the assurance that "having some won't hurt just this once." Anyone who continues to pressure you is not really a friend, or at the very least does not care about your best interests. Remember that you are following the Princeton Plan because you want to lose weight and keep it off while following the healthiest possible long-term diet. Your goal is *not* to return to your former high-fat, high-salt, high-sugar diet, but rather to achieve a permanent and healthful change in your eating habits. Eating those unhealthful dishes on occasion will only perpetuate your addiction to the foods that keep you fat. (For more information on sugar addiction, see pages 240–241).

Holidays also combine an abundance of tempting unhealthful foods with pressure to eat and overeat. If you are responsible for preparing your holiday meal, follow the guidelines for adapting family recipes on page 219. For example, serve turkey without the skin, prepare clear, defatted broth instead of gravy, make dressing from whole-wheat bread or grain, and moisten it with broth rather than pan drippings; serve steamed vegetables garnished with lemon; cut visible fat off the roast or ham before serving.

If you are having a holiday dinner elsewhere, follow the guidelines for eating out, and avoid fatty and rich foods. There will always be something you can eat; or you can bring your own grain-and-vegetable side dish.

FOLLOWING THE PRINCETON PLAN ON
THE ROAD

Don't use travel—either for vacation or business—as an excuse to stop following the Princeton Plan. Continue to observe our guidelines when eating in restaurants, or use room service—many hotel kitchens will prepare foods cooked to your specifications for delivery to your room. Another strategy is to find a nearby market or deli and buy some low-fat yogurt and fruit or vegetables to take back to your room. Or, you can take packets of the Princeton Plan powdered drink with you (see page 68).

When you make your airline reservations, request a low-fat, low-salt meal. Most major airlines will comply with a wide variety of special dietary requests. Or bring your own healthful sandwich and fruit.

Finally, don't neglect your three-part exercise plan. As a matter of fact, exercising regularly can help you more quickly overcome jet lag or stiffness caused by sitting for long periods in a cramped airplane seat.

When you're on vacation, sightseeing is a great way to get acquainted with a new place and get your aerobics in at the same time. Just remember to walk at least 20 continual minutes at a pace fast enough to get your heart into the training zone. If you have progressed to more vigorous exercise, check with the hotel front desk for nearby jogging routes. Some hotels even offer exercise trails, and increasing numbers of hotels provide gyms and swimming pools for the convenience of their fitness-minded patrons.

Remember that the Princeton Plan is designed to help you lose weight *and* to ensure that you live the healthiest possible life-style. It may not be as "easy" to live the Princeton way as it is to be a couch potato who never moves from the tube except to open another pack of corn chips. But once you have made the Princeton Plan a part of your life, we think you will feel so good and have so much extra energy that you won't even want to think about returning to your bad old habits.

QUESTIONS PEOPLE ASK ABOUT THE PRINCETON PLAN

I sometimes find it hard to eat everything allowed, especially on the high-calorie days. Is it all right to skip some exchanges?

All parts of the Princeton Plan have been scientifically designed to help you lose weight steadily without the "plateau" that occurs on other diets as your metabolism slows. By alternating low-carbohydrate, low-calorie days with high-carbohydrate, high-calorie days, we combine the benefits of the two most common diets—the high-protein, high-fat diets, and the high-carbohydrate diets—but without any of the disadvantages of those regimens. When averaged over the two-day dietary intake, the Princeton Plan meets the government's requirements for a balanced diet while at the same time stimulating metabolism.

Remember that unlike traditional diets, the Princeton Plan provides *complete* nutrition. All foods listed in the daily exchanges contribute to that nutrition and should be eaten. Perhaps you are so used to feeling hungry on a diet that you are just feeling guilty about having so much to eat.

Is it necessary to take all the supplements?

Any diet that contains fewer than 1800 calories is very unlikely to meet the RDA requirements for all nutrients. This goes for the Princeton Plan as well. In addition, exercise requires extra nutrients, primarily the antioxidants needed to combat the free radicals produced by physical activity. Certain other supplements are necessary to stimulate thermogenesis (see page 99 for details).

Remember that none of the suggested supplements is toxic at the levels we recommend.

Can I just go on the diet and not exercise?

No. While you might lose weight for a while, eventually your metabolism will slow down. Any diet that does not include a realistic exercise program is doomed to failure.

Can I just exercise and not go on the diet?

Perhaps. But only if your normal diet is already a healthy, balanced one, relying on whole, unprocessed foods as we recommend in this book.

I want to take up swimming for my aerobic exercise. But I read somewhere that swimmers don't lose weight. Is that true?

In the studies showing that swimmers don't lose (or gain) weight, no attempt was made to record what the subjects ate. Thus, a big part of the energy-balance equation—energy intake—was not even addressed. The researchers felt that swimmers probably have a tendency to eat more because water carries body heat away more quickly than air, thus stimulating appetite to compensate for the calories lost. No matter what kind of exercise you do, you must regulate your calorie intake when you're trying to lose weight. As long as you combine the Princeton Eating Plan with your swimming program, you will lose weight.

Is it possible to lose fat from particular areas of the body?

Alas for those with less-than-perfect figures, the idea of "spot reduction" is a myth. Aerobic exercise and diet combined will help you lose fat, but it will come from all over your body, not just the part that is being exercised. Walkers and bikers will lose fat from their arms as well as from their legs and hips.

By following the strength-building part of the Princeton Exercise Program, you can *reshape* particular areas of your body. Strong abdominal muscles, for example, act like a corset, giving you a firm, flat belly, while weak abdominals allow your internal organs to push against your abdominal wall and make you look flabby. Similarly, exercising the chest muscles can help to produce a high, firm bustline.

How can I tell if I'm getting more brown fat?

At present there is really no way to measure your brown fat. Certain laboratory techniques, including infrared thermography and the measurement of certain enzymes, have been used on test subjects, but these methods are not practical for most people. Autopsies have shown increased brown fat in Finnish outdoor workers and Korean pearl divers. The best way to know if you are turning on your brown fat is to observe a slow, steady loss of weight with no plateau effect.

I like to lift weights. Is aerobic exercise really necessary too?

Aerobic exercise is essential for weight loss. The main fuel for slow aerobic exercise is fat, and fat is what you are trying to get rid of. The main fuel for anaerobic exercises, including weight training, is glycogen (stored sugar).

When I gain weight, I always put it on in my hips, while my best friend gains in her stomach and upper body. Why is this?

The pattern of fat distribution is probably determined by genetic factors and cannot be changed. Recent research has demonstrated that there are two types of obesity: abdominal, or upper-body obesity, and gluteal-femoral, or lower-body obesity. Interestingly, those with upper-body fat have relatively *large* fat cells, while those with the lower-body type have a relatively high *number* of fat cells.

It may be harder for those with lower-body obesity to lose weight, but the upper-body pattern is associated with more health risks, including diabetes, hypertension, and heart disease. No matter where you carry the fat on your body, the healthiest thing you can do is to follow the Princeton Plan and reduce it to lower levels.

Can the number of fat cells be reduced once they have formed?

The only way to remove fat cells is through liposuction, a somewhat controversial surgical procedure.

My brother is not overweight, but he is out of shape. Can the Princeton Plan help him?

Yes. It is essentially a life-style plan that can be followed for the rest of your life. If your brother does not need to lose weight, he should increase the number of food exchanges that he eats.

I've been following the Princeton Plan faithfully, and I feel better and my clothes are looser, but I'm not losing much weight. What should I do?

One to three pounds a week is a reasonable weight-loss goal for most people. However, you may need to reduce the "core number" of calories that you alternate your menus around (see Appendix A).

On the other hand, if your clothes are looser, you are probably losing fat and replacing it with muscle, which weighs more than fat but takes up less space. Remember that the Princeton Plan is *not* a crash diet; rather, it is a sensible eating and exercise plan that you can follow for your entire life.

I like the diet but the beans give me gas. Is there anything I can do about this?

Cooked beans, a valuable source of vegetable protein, are the most potent producer of gas known to man. The gas is caused by bacteria in the large intestine which ferment indigestible parts of the bean. To compound the problem, the raw starch in inadequately cooked beans can cause even more gas.

Fortunately, there is a remedy at hand. First, make certain that all beans are thoroughly cooked. Then, if you still have problems with excess gas, soak beans for several hours before cooking and *discard the soaking water.* Then cook as usual in fresh water. Although some nutrients will be lost, the loss won't be significant, and the beans should no longer cause flatulence.

Should I exercise when I'm feeling sick?

If you just feel a little under the weather, you may be surprised to find that your exercise routine will awaken your body and make you feel better. If, on the other hand, you are too sick to go to work or are running a fever, it's better to just relax and drink plenty of fluids. If you must stop your aerobic routine for several days because of illness, remember to start at a slightly lower level when you return to it.

The Princeton Plan sounds great, but whenever I go on a diet my hands and feet get cold. Will that happen on the Princeton Plan?

It's possible that you have Reynaud's syndrome, a condition in which small arteries become restricted in response to cold, resulting in painfully cold extremities. The problem can get worse when calories are restricted. New studies show, however, that this syndrome is helped by supplements of the essential fatty acids found in fish oils. Since the Princeton Plan is generous in these nutrients, it is possible that you will suffer no symptoms as long as you follow the guidelines.

I am milk-intolerant. Can I still follow the Princeton Plan?

The majority of adults in the world have difficulty digesting lactose, the sugar found in milk, because they are deficient in the enzyme lactase. This is especially true for blacks and orientals. It is now possible to buy milk that has been treated with lactase ("Lactaid"); most people find that this product causes no problems. You can also buy Lactaid tablets and drops in the drug store to add to milk. If you simply do not like milk, you can satisfy your dairy requirements with other products, such as yogurt, which can be digested by many people with lactose intolerance. It can also help to take milk products along with other foods.

I am a strict vegetarian. Can I follow the Princeton Plan?

It is more difficult to get all the necessary nutrients on a strictly vegetarian diet but, with planning, such a regimen can be nutritious and healthful. See Appendix B for a vegetarian eating plan.

THE PRINCETON SUPER PLAN: SPECIAL STRATEGIES AND SUPPLEMENTS

FOLLOWING the basic Princeton Plan will help you achieve your goal of lasting weight loss and should help you feel healthier and achieve a firmer body. You needn't, in fact, do anything more than you are already doing. However, if you want to increase your thermogenesis even more, speed weight loss, and increase the effectiveness of the exercise you are doing, you may want to try some of the suggestions in this chapter. Some involve taking supplements for specific purposes; others are strategies for increasing the benefits of exercise. Remember that not all suggestions are for everyone and that you needn't adopt any of them if you don't want to.

SUPER PLAN EXERCISE

The basic Princeton Exercise Plan is designed to speed up your metabolism and produce thermogenesis; the super plan can increase both of these benefits, enabling you to burn calories at an even greater rate. Most of the following tips work directly to increase thermogenesis, which, you may recall, is produced in response to food intake and cold temperatures. Cold temperatures actually turn on BAT, and recent studies show that temperatures as high as 71.6 degrees Fahrenheit are in fact low enough to stimulate cold-induced thermogenesis. Furthermore, these effects are enhanced when exercise is added. To take advantage of the exercise and cold connection, try the following:

- **Whenever possible, exercise in a cool environment.** This should be easy in the winter—simply walk or jog outdoors and open a window while doing your strength-building exercises. In hot weather, try exercising in front of a fan or air conditioner; if possible, do your aerobic exercise in an air-conditioned mall or health club. If you're not always able to exercise in cool temperatures, however, don't worry: Remember the many benefits that exercise is conferring no matter what the temperature.

- **Wear cool, loose-fitting clothes during exercise.** When working out in the cold it is better to underdress slightly than to overdress; your effort will soon warm you up. If you're jogging or walking outside in very cold weather, dress in layers that you can take off one by one and tie around your waist as you warm up. (*Note:* In severe weather, it's better to bundle up, wearing a hat and protecting your extremities against frostbite. Petroleum jelly can help protect your face and hands from the biting, chapping effects of a cold wind.)

- **Take cool showers or baths both before and after exercise.**

- **If convenient, apply a cold towel over the back of your neck and/or lower back while exercising.** The cold will directly affect your BAT, especially concentrated in these areas, and turn it on. If you are handy with a needle, you might create a "thermogenic jacket" with special pockets to carry cold packs over these areas.

- **Be aware that cold can stimulate appetite**, and guard against the temptation to overeat after a cool workout. Studies indicate that nondieting swimmers who exercise in cold water have a tendency to gain weight.

- **Wear your lost weight.** As you lose weight, your metabolism will slow down somewhat with each pound you lose. To keep your body's fires burning at maximum, try wearing or carrying weight packs to simulate that lost avoirdupois. For example, after your first loss of 5 pounds, place 2½-pound ankle weights on each leg. To avoid injury, however, *do not* do aerobics or other exercises while wearing weights; simply wear them around the house. Also, never wear more than a total of 10 pounds.

PEAK PERFORMANCE

The concept of **peak performance**—pushing yourself to a maximum physical effort—is well known to trained athletes. Surprisingly, studies show that nonathletes can use the same principles to make exercise more effective. In fact, peak performance during exercise can markedly increase strength and aerobic fitness.

The most common way of achieving peak performance is to use interval training. This training method, long advocated by track coaches, involves pushing beyond what is comfortable and then resting briefly before pushing again. The result is increased ability to use oxygen and a rapid growth in aerobic capacity and strength. Even if you are not interested in further improving your exercise capability, studies indicate that peak performance efforts stimulate growth hormone (see page 237), which reduces fat and increases lean tissue, thus upping metabolism.

In an article in *Health* magazine, author Joan Liffert describes a study of ordinary nonathletic women who exercised on stationary bicycles. Volunteers who spent only 12 minutes a session at interval work improved their cardiovascular health as much as did women who "biked" at a slow steady pace for 20 minutes. Another experiment, using aerobic dancers, confirmed these findings, demonstrating that after twelve weeks the interval-trained dancers increased their aerobic fitness almost twice as much as exercisers who worked at a slower, steady pace.

Not only is interval training more efficient than slow and steady exercise, it can also be more pleasant, because you're not always doing the same thing in the same way.

If you want to incorporate interval training into your exercise routine, wait until you have reached the maintenance level of your aerobic exercise, then simply add one or more intense, all-out efforts of a few seconds to a minute or so. Walk especially fast, for example, then rest for at least the same amount of time by walking at your normal pace or even slower. If you jog for exercise, try sprints. The intervals needn't be done in any systematic way. In fact, some experts think the best way to incorporate this type of training into your routine is to adopt the Scandinavian system of *fartlek,* or "speed-play," in which you vary the pace on an irregular basis, whenever you feel like it.

SUPPLEMENTS THAT TURN UP
THERMOGENESIS

A common myth for years was that athletes need extra protein for optimal performance. Today we know that this isn't true; that, in fact, the primary fuels used in physical endeavors are fat and carbohydrate. Nevertheless, anyone who works out should be sure to get supplemental nutrition, principally the antioxidants we recommend in the Princeton Eating Plan, to eliminate the excess free radicals that are produced by exercise.

There are also a number of other supplements that have been proven in some studies to enhance athletic performance and/or to increase thermogenesis. We do not recommend that you take all or even any of these, but you may find some of them useful additions to the basic Princeton Plan. Except where noted, all are safe when taken in the quantities indicated.

Note: There is always a possibility of idiosyncratic responses when you begin to take unaccustomed nutrients. If you notice any adverse physical reactions, such as diarrhea or nausea, or psychological reactions, such as sleeplessness or depression, discontinue any *new* supplements and consult with a doctor or nutritionist before resuming the supplement or supplements.

GAMMA-LINOLENIC ACID

Gamma-linolenic acid is a metabolite of linoleic acid and an important precursor of the "good" prostaglandin PGE1. The exciting news about gamma-linolenic acid is that a number of studies have shown that it causes some overweight people to lose weight *without dieting* or otherwise restricting calories. This effect is thought to be especially pronounced for those whose tendency to gain weight is inherited. Although not everything is known about its weight-loss-enhancing mechanism, gamma-linolenic acid is believed to increase brown fat and stimulate thermogenesis.

In addition to turning up thermogenesis, gamma-linolenic acid has also been found (again, as a precursor to prostaglandins) to be beneficial in a number of disorders, from premenstrual syndrome and menstrual cramps to atherosclerosis, high blood pressure, and elevated cholesterol.

Gamma-linolenic acid is found in Evening Primrose Oil, borage, and black-currant-seed oil. (*Note:* Gamma-linolenic acid should be taken with meals, and, for maximum effectiveness, it must be taken with the prostaglandin cofactors zinc, magnesium, and vitamins B_6 and B_3, all of which are included in our list of recommended supplements on pages 99 to 101.)

CARNITINE

Carnitine, an amino acid responsible for transporting fat molecules for burning within the cell, is found primarily in red meat, but it may also be taken as a supplement to increase thermogenesis. Fats *cannot* be burned as fuel in the absence of carnitine; if your diet does not include at least some red meat, you should take supplements to aid in weight loss, or eat tempeh, a fermented soy product that is the main vegetarian source of this nutrient. As a supplement, take one 600-mg. capsule of carnitine twice daily.

COENZYME Q-10

Coenzyme Q-10, which is present in all human tissues, plays a key role in each cell's production of energy. In addition, it has been shown to stimulate the immune system, and it acts as an antioxidant within the cells, protecting cell structures from free radicals produced when fuel is burned for energy. Coenzyme Q-10 has been used for years in Japan to treat a wide variety of disorders, including heart disease and high blood pressure. In recent years, studies have shown that Coenzyme Q-10, taken as a supplement, also speeds up the metabolism and increases the burning of fat.

Of particular interest is a study determining that as many as 50 percent of overweight people are deficient in Coenzyme Q-10; when given supplements in conjunction with a diet, volunteers lost weight at a far greater rate than other subjects who dieted but did not receive supplementation.

Even in large amounts, Coenzyme Q-10 is not toxic. To aid in weight loss, we recommend taking 30–60 mg. a day, with meals (the supplement comes in 10- and 30-mg. capsules). For maintenance and disease prevention, we recommend 10 to 30 mg. a day.

GLUCOSE TOLERANCE FACTOR

Glucose tolerance factor, composed partly of organic chromium, is essential for proper use of insulin, which itself, as we have noted, is essential in glucose regulation, fat storage, and thermogenesis. The type and quantity of foods commonly produced and eaten in the United States may predispose us to low tissue concentrations of chromium, leading to impaired glucose tolerance, and in some individuals a craving for sweets. Studies have shown that diabetics taking chromium supplements were able to reduce their daily dosage of insulin. Another study on elderly volunteers showed that supplements of glucose tolerance factor (in brewer's yeast) led to normal glucose tolerance.

As a supplement, take 200 mcgs. of chromium daily with dinner on the high-carbohydrate day. Note that the Princeton Plan P.M. Formula (page 101) contains 200 mcg. of chromium.

BRANCHED-CHAIN AMINO ACIDS

Branched-chain amino acids, which are essential to human health, include the nutrients valine, isoleucine, and leucine. These substances stimulate the synthesis of protein and inhibit its breakdown, promoting muscle growth and maintenance and thus leading to increased metabolic rate.

For peak uptake by the muscles, these amino acids should be taken on the low-carbohydrate day, 60 to 90 minutes after a workout. Recommended dosage: 1000 mg l-isoleucine; 1500 mg. l-leucine; and 1250 mg. l-valine.

GROWTH HORMONE

Growth hormone, produced by the pituitary gland, encourages the body to build muscle and burn fat. As we get older, natural production of growth hormone slows down. Luckily, through supplementation and other strategies, we can increase our body's production of this important substance, leading to a higher muscle-to-fat ratio and thus a higher metabolic rate.

Growth hormone is produced in response to a number of stimuli, among them sleep and exercise itself, especially peak-performance exercise (see page 233). In addition, certain amino acids stimulate the pituitary gland to produce and release this hormone.

To stimulate the formation of growth hormone, take 100 mg. of l-arginine with 500 mg. of l-ornithine on an empty stomach at bedtime on the low-carbohydrate day.

To stimulate the release of growth hormone, take 1200 mg. each of l-arginine and l-lysine on an empty stomach at bedtime on the low-carbohydrate day.

HISTIDINE

Histidine, an amino acid, encourages the formation of the "good" prostaglandin PGE1. In addition, histidine is the precursor of histamine, which has been shown in studies to suppress food consumption and thus lead to weight loss.

TRYPTOPHAN

Tryptophan, another amino acid, helps speed weight loss in more than one way. Like arginine, ornithine, and lysine, it has been shown to stimulate production of growth hormone, leading to increased muscle growth. In addition, it stimulates formation of serotonin, a neurotransmitter that increases BAT. There is also evidence that tryptophan can decrease appetite and especially reduce any craving for carbohydrates.

As a supplement, take 500 mg. of tryptophan two or three times during the high-calorie, high-carbohydrate day, to curb appetite and control carbohydrate craving. (Begin with the lower dose; if no effect is noted, increase gradually.) Take it *with* a carbohydrate food in the between-meal snack or on an empty stomach. Trytophan is most effective when taken at the time of day when cravings usually occur; for most people, that is usually late afternoon and after dinner.

SUPPLEMENTS THAT TURN ON BAT

PHENYLALANINE AND TYROSINE

Phenylalanine and tyrosine amino acids are converted into norepinephrine, which stimulates BAT. Artificial sweeteners made with aspartame may contribute small amounts of phenylalanine to the diet. Some studies suggest that aspartame in large doses may cause mood changes in laboratory rats, so care is advised in its use. Phenylalanine should not be used in patients with PKU (phenylketonuria).

Phenylalanine should be taken on the low-carbohydrate day, in a dose of 500 mg., morning and night, either with main meals or snacks.

GAMMA-AMINOBUTYRIC ACID

Gamma-aminobutyric acid (GABA), an amino acid that serves as a neurotransmitter, is believed to be involved in the regulation of food intake and body weight. Rats fed supplements of GABA eat less and lose weight; it is thought that GABA increases sympathetic stimulation of BAT.

To increase GABA, take l-glutamine (a precursor of GABA) in a dose of 500 mg. morning and evening on the high-carbohydrate day, since its effects are greater when the diet is low in protein.

METABOLIC STIMULANTS

EPHEDRA

Ephedra, a Chinese herb that has been used as a stimulant for centuries, increases metabolism by stimulating the sympathetic nervous system to secrete norepinephrine (for details, see chapter 3). Several studies have shown that a single dose of the active ingredient—ephedrine—stimulates thermogenesis and that with continued usage the metabolic rate continues to increase. Ephedrine also directly stimulates the burning of fat.

Note: No one should take supplements of ephedra without medical supervision. Although centuries of use have established the tea's basic safety, some people find it can make them very nervous and jittery. Remember that ephedra is a stimulant, so it should not be drunk late in the day or at night. When taken in larger doses it can cause dizziness and insomnia. Finally, *do not* use this substance without your doctor's advice if you have high blood pressure, heart or thyroid disease, or diabetes. Ephedra should *never* be given to children under the age of three or drunk by pregnant or nursing women.

CAFFEINE

A common stimulant, found naturally in coffee and chocolate (and added to many soft drinks and over-the-counter medications), caffeine can actually increase your resting metabolic rate. Studies have shown that for many people a dose of caffeine (in coffee) *before* exercise can improve the ability to burn fat as a fuel during exercise, thus diminishing fatigue and increasing endurance, as well as enhancing weight loss. This effect of caffeine seems to be enhanced when combined with ephedra.

There are a number of drawbacks to regular caffeine consumption, however, including the possibility of nervousness, irritability, and insomnia. Anyone who experiences any of these symptoms with relatively low doses of caffeine (one to two cups of coffee a day) is probably hypersensitive to caffeine and shouldn't use it at all. Caffeine should not be used by women with cystic breast disease, and pregnant and nursing women should also limit consumption.

A better bet for many people is theophylline (see below).

THEOPHYLLINE

This substance, found in regular (nonherbal) tea, is, like caffeine, a member of a class of stimulants called *methylxanthines*. Like caffeine, theophylline can help increase thermogenesis and the burning of fat during exercise; it also enhances the thermogenic effect of ephedra. For a thermogenic effect, drink 1 to 3 cups of tea a day.

Tea causes less gastric upset and other symptoms than coffee, although it shouldn't be used by pregnant women or women with cystic breast disease.

DEALING WITH SUGAR ADDICTION

Unlike many traditional diets, the Princeton Plan does not allow occasional refined-sugar "treats," nor does it encourage the consumption of artificial sweeteners. Through psychological as well as physiological mechanisms, all such sweets preserve an abnormal craving for sugar.

Fructose, the sugar found in fruits, is digested more slowly than sucrose (table sugar) and does not cause a steep rise in blood sugar (followed by a release of large amounts of insulin, and then a sudden, reactive drop in blood sugar). If you must have extra sweets, it's far better to "overeat" fruits, which contain, in addition to fructose, fiber, minerals, and vitamins. Note that the Princeton Plan P.M. Formula (page 101) contains 200 mcg. of chromium. Chromium has been shown to decrease sugar cravings in some individuals.

Dr. Gary Evans, a research scientist working with the U.S. Department of Agriculture, has demonstrated in two recent studies the ability of chromium picolinate to increase lean body mass (muscle) and decrease total body fat. Picolinic acid is derived from the amino acid tryptophan. The combination of picolinic acid with chromium appears to magnify the tissue-building properties of insulin. It is noteworthy that in the Princeton Plan Formulas, chromium, as picolinate, is used.

Once you have reached your goal weight, you may feel that you can go back to eating sugary desserts again, but we urge you to resist the temptation; for many failed dieters the reintroduction of gooey desserts is the beginning of a regain of lost weight. "It's like one drink for an alcoholic," says a health professional who finally overcame a years-long sugar addiction. "If I'd have just one chocolate I'd be back bingeing on candy." After many months of abstaining from sweets this woman eventually overcame her addiction and is now able to have "just one" on widely separated occasions.

APPENDIX A.
CUSTOMIZING THE PRINCETON
PLAN TO YOUR OWN
METABOLISM

IN order to plan your own menus, you need to know the caloric intake at which you lose weight. We will call this the **core number**. Women usually lose weight at 1200 calories per day and men at 1500 calories. If you are very overweight and/or have yo-yoed a number of times, you may need to choose a lower core number. If, on the other hand, you are very active and normally eat 2500 or more calories a day, you may need to choose a higher core number. Or you may simply calculate your present caloric intake, lower it by a few hundred calories, and use that as your core number.

To avoid the plateau effect of dieting, the Princeton Plan alternates low- and high-calorie days, which deviate from the core number of calories by approximately 30 percent. Thus, for a dieter whose core number is 1800 calories, the daily menus would alternate between 1500 calories on the low-calorie day and 2000 calories on the high-calorie day, averaging approximately 1800 calories a day.

The box on page 244 shows a range of core numbers and the corresponding calories to be eaten on alternating days.

In addition to alternating caloric intake, the Princeton Plan alternates nutrient intake to stimulate the metabolic rate. On the lower-calorie day, 45% of the calories are from carbohydrate, 25% are from

CORE NUMBERS AND ALTERNATE CALORIE ALLOWANCES

Core Number of Calories	Calories for Alternating Days
800	600–900
900	700–1000
1000	800–1100
1100	900–1200
1200	1000–1400
1300	1100–1500
1400	1200–1600
1500	1200–1700
1600	1300–1800
1700	1400–1900
1800	1500–2000
1900	1600–2200
2000	1700–2300
2100	1800–2400
2200	1900–2500

protein, and 30% are from fat. On the higher-calorie day, 65 percent of the calories are from carbohydrate, 15 percent are from protein, and 20 percent are from fat.

In the following pages are a number of daily meal plans, for a wide range of alternating low- and high-calorie days. To use them, simply turn to the exchange lists on pages 134–142 and choose exchanges from the lists for the foods allowed in each menu block.

If you prefer to make your own menu plans, use the two tables on pages 245–246, which provide the food exchanges to be used on the low- and high-calorie days. For example, if your alternating numbers are 800 and 1100, use the food exchanges opposite 800 on the low-calorie table and the food exchanges opposite 1100 on the high-calorie table. Then turn to the food-exchange lists starting on page 134 and fill in your daily menu plan.

TABLE OF EXCHANGES

Low-Calorie, Low-Carbohydrate Day
25% Protein, 45% Carbohydrate, 30% Fat

Calories	Milk	Veg	Fruit	Grain or Bread	Meat	Fat
600	1	2	2	1	3	2
700	1	2	2	2	4	2
800	1	3	2	2	5	2
900	1	3	2	3	5	3
1000	1	3	2	3	6	4
1100	1	3	2	4	6	4
1200	1	3	2	5	7	4
1300	2	3	3	4	7	4
1400	2	4	3	5	7	5
1500	2	4	3	5	8	6
1600	2	4	3	6	8	6
1700	2	4	3	7	8	7
1800	3	4	3	7	8	7
1900	3	4	4	7	9	7
2000	3	4	4	8	9	8

TABLE OF EXCHANGES

High-Calorie, High-Carbohydrate Day
15% Protein, 65% Carbohydrate, 20% Fat

Calories	Milk	Veg	Fruit	Grain or Bread	Meat	Fat
900	1	3	2	6	0	4
1000	1	3	3	6	0	5
1100	1	3	2	8	0	5
1200	1	4	2	9	0	5
1300	2	3	3	9	0	6
1400	2	3	3	10	0	6
1500	2	4	3	10	0	7
1600	2	4	4	11	0	7
1700	2	4	4	12	0	7
1800	3	4	4	12	0	8
1900	3	4	4	13	0	8
2000	3	4	4	14	0	9
2100	3	5	4	15	0	9
2200	3	5	5	15	0	10
2300	4	5	5	15	0	10
2400	4	5	5	16	0	10
2500	4	5	5	16	0	11

600-Calorie, Low-Calorie, Low-Carbohydrate Day

Breakfast

    1 fruit exchange   _____

    1 milk exchange   _____

Morning Snack

Lunch

    1 meat exchange   _____

    1 veg exchange   _____

    1 fat exchange   _____

Afternoon Snack

    1 bread exchange   _____

Dinner

    2 meat exchanges   _____

    1 veg exchange   _____

    1 fat exchange   _____

Evening Snack

    1 fruit exchange   _____

Milk	Veg	Fruit	Bread	Meat	Fat
1	2	2	1	3	2

700-Calorie, Low-Calorie, Low-Carbohydrate Day

Breakfast

    ½ bread exchange   _____

    ½ fat exchange   _____

    ½ fruit exchange   _____

    1 milk exchange   _____

Morning Snack

    ½ bread exchange   _____

    ½ fruit exchange   _____

Lunch

    2 meat exchanges   _____

    ½ bread exchange   _____

    1 veg exchange   _____

    ½ fat exchange   _____

Afternoon Snack

    ½ fruit exchange   _____

Dinner

    2 meat exchanges   _____

    ½ bread exchange   _____

    1 veg exchange   _____

    1 fat exchange   _____

Evening Snack

    ½ fruit exchange   _____

Milk	Veg	Fruit	Bread	Meat	Fat
1	2	2	2	4	2

800-Calorie, Low-Calorie, Low-Carbohydrate Day

Breakfast

    ½ bread exchange   _____
    ½ fat exchange   _____
    ½ fruit exchange   _____
    ½ milk exchange   _____

Morning Snack

    ½ bread exchange   _____
    ½ fruit exchange   _____

Lunch

    2½ meat exchanges   _____
    ½ bread exchange   _____
    1½ veg exchanges   _____
    ½ fat exchange   _____

Afternoon Snack

    ½ fruit exchange   _____

Dinner

    2½ meat exchanges   _____
    ½ bread exchange   _____
    1½ veg exchanges   _____
    1 fat exchange   _____

Evening Snack

    ½ fruit exchange   _____
    ½ milk exchange   _____

Milk	Veg	Fruit	Bread	Meat	Fat
1	3	2	2	5	2

900-Calorie, Low-Calorie, Low-Carbohydrate Day

Breakfast

    ½ bread exchange   _____

    ½ fat exchange   _____

    ½ fruit exchange   _____

    ½ milk exchange   _____

Morning Snack

    ½ bread exchange   _____

    ½ fruit exchange   _____

Lunch

    2½ meat exchanges   _____

    1 bread exchange   _____

    1½ veg exchanges   _____

    1½ fat exchanges   _____

Afternoon Snack

    ½ fruit exchange   _____

Dinner

    2½ meat exchanges   _____

    1 bread exchange   _____

    1½ veg exchanges   _____

    1 fat exchange   _____

Evening Snack

    ½ fruit exchange   _____

    ½ milk exchange   _____

Milk	Veg	Fruit	Bread	Meat	Fat
1	3	2	3	5	3

1000-Calorie, Low-Calorie, Low-Carbohydrate Day

Breakfast

    ½ bread exchange   _____
    1 fat exchange   _____
    ½ fruit exchange   _____
    ½ milk exchange   _____

Morning Snack

    ½ bread exchange   _____
    ½ fruit exchange   _____

Lunch

    3 meat exchanges   _____
    1 bread exchange   _____
    1½ veg exchanges   _____
    1½ fat exchanges   _____

Afternoon Snack

    ½ fruit exchange   _____

Dinner

    3 meat exchanges   _____
    1 bread exchange   _____
    1½ veg exchanges   _____
    1½ fat exchanges   _____

Evening Snack

    ½ fruit exchange   _____
    ½ milk exchange   _____

Milk	Veg	Fruit	Bread	Meat	Fat
1	3	2	3	6	4

1100-Calorie, Low-Calorie, Low-Carbohydrate Day

Breakfast

    1 bread exchange   _____

    1 fat exchange   _____

    ½ fruit exchange   _____

    ½ milk exchange   _____

Morning Snack

    1 bread exchange   _____

    ½ fruit exchange   _____

Lunch

    3 meat exchanges   _____

    1 bread exchange   _____

    1½ veg exchanges   _____

    1½ fat exchanges   _____

Afternoon Snack

    ½ fruit exchange   _____

Dinner

    3 meat exchanges   _____

    1 bread exchange   _____

    1½ veg exchanges   _____

    1½ fat exchanges   _____

Evening Snack

    ½ fruit exchange   _____

    ½ milk exchange   _____

Milk	Veg	Fruit	Bread	Meat	Fat
1	3	2	4	6	4

1200-Calorie, Low-Calorie, Low-Carbohydrate Day

Breakfast

    1 bread exchange   _____
    1 fat exchange   _____
    ½ fruit exchange   _____
    ½ milk exchange   _____

Morning Snack

    1 bread exchange   _____
    ½ fruit exchange   _____

Lunch

    3½ meat exchanges   _____
    1½ bread exchanges   _____
    1½ veg exchanges   _____
    1½ fat exchanges   _____

Afternoon Snack

    ½ fruit exchange   _____

Dinner

    3½ meat exchanges   _____
    1½ bread exchanges   _____
    1½ veg exchanges   _____
    1½ fat exchanges   _____

Evening Snack

    ½ fruit exchange   _____
    ½ milk exchange   _____

Milk	Veg	Fruit	Bread	Meat	Fat
1	3	2	5	7	4

1300-Calorie, Low-Calorie, Low-Carbohydrate Day

Breakfast

    1 bread exchange   _____

    1 fat exchange   _____

    ½ fruit exchange   _____

    1 milk exchange   _____

Morning Snack

    1 bread exchange   _____

    ½ fruit exchange   _____

Lunch

    3½ meat exchanges   _____

    1 bread exchange   _____

    1½ veg exchanges   _____

    1½ fat exchanges   _____

Afternoon Snack

    1 fruit exchange   _____

Dinner

    3½ meat exchanges   _____

    1 bread exchange   _____

    1½ veg exchanges   _____

    1½ fat exchanges   _____

Evening Snack

    1 fruit exchange   _____

    1 milk exchange   _____

Milk	Veg	Fruit	Bread	Meat	Fat
2	3	3	4	7	4

1400-Calorie, Low-Calorie, Low-Carbohydrate Day

Breakfast

    1 bread exchange   _____
    1 fat exchange   _____
    ½ fruit exchange   _____
    1 milk exchange   _____

Morning Snack

    1 bread exchange   _____
    ½ fruit exchange   _____

Lunch

    3½ meat exchanges   _____
    1½ bread exchanges   _____
    2 veg exchanges   _____
    2 fat exchanges   _____

Afternoon Snack

    1 fruit exchange   _____

Dinner

    3½ meat exchanges   _____
    1½ bread exchanges   _____
    2 veg exchanges   _____
    2 fat exchanges   _____

Evening Snack

    1 fruit exchange   _____
    1 milk exchange   _____

Milk	Veg	Fruit	Bread	Meat	Fat
2	4	3	5	7	5

1500-Calorie, Low-Calorie, Low-Carbohydrate Day

Breakfast

    1 bread exchange   _____

    1 fat exchange   _____

    ½ fruit exchange   _____

    1 milk exchange   _____

Morning Snack

    1 bread exchange   _____

    ½ fruit exchange   _____

Lunch

    4 meat exchanges   _____

    1½ bread exchanges   _____

    2 veg exchanges   _____

    2½ fat exchanges   _____

Afternoon Snack

    1 fruit exchange   _____

Dinner

    4 meat exchanges   _____

    1½ bread exchanges   _____

    2 veg exchanges   _____

    2½ fat exchanges   _____

Evening Snack

    1 fruit exchange   _____

    1 milk exchange   _____

Milk	Veg	Fruit	Bread	Meat	Fat
2	4	3	5	8	6

1600-Calorie, Low-Calorie, Low-Carbohydrate Day

Breakfast

    1 bread exchange   _____

    1 fat exchange   _____

    1 fruit exchange   _____

    ½ milk exchange   _____

Morning Snack

    1 fruit exchange   _____

Lunch

    3 meat exchanges   _____

    2 bread exchanges   _____

    1 veg exchange   _____

    2½ fat exchanges   _____

    ½ milk exchange   _____

Afternoon Snack

    ½ bread exchange   _____

Dinner

    5 meat exchanges   _____

    2 bread exchanges   _____

    3 veg exchanges   _____

    2½ fat exchanges   _____

Evening Snack

    ½ bread exchange   _____

    1 fruit exchange   _____

Milk	Veg	Fruit	Bread	Meat	Fat
2	4	3	6	8	6

1700-Calorie, Low-Calorie, Low-Carbohydrate Day

Breakfast

    1½ bread exchanges   _____

    1½ fat exchanges   _____

    1 fruit exchange   _____

    ½ milk exchange   _____

Morning Snack

    1 fruit exchange   _____

Lunch

    3 meat exchanges   _____

    2½ bread exchanges   _____

    1 veg exchange   _____

    2½ fat exchanges   _____

    ½ milk exchange   _____

Afternoon Snack

    ½ bread exchange   _____

Dinner

    5 meat exchanges   _____

    2 bread exchanges   _____

    3 veg exchanges   _____

    3 fat exchanges   _____

    1 milk exchange   _____

Evening Snack

    ½ bread exchange   _____

    1 fruit exchange   _____

Milk	Veg	Fruit	Bread	Meat	Fat
2	4	3	7	8	7

1800-Calorie, Low-Calorie, Low-Carbohydrate Day

Breakfast

    1 ½ bread exchanges   _____

    1 ½ fat exchanges   _____

    1 fruit exchange   _____

    1 milk exchange   _____

Morning Snack

    1 fruit exchange   _____

Lunch

    3 meat exchanges   _____

    2 ½ bread exchanges   _____

    1 veg exchange   _____

    2 ½ fat exchanges   _____

    1 milk exchange   _____

Afternoon Snack

    ½ bread exchange   _____

Dinner

    5 meat exchanges   _____

    2 bread exchanges   _____

    3 veg exchanges   _____

    3 fat exchanges   _____

    1 milk exchange   _____

Evening Snack

    ½ bread exchange   _____

    1 fruit exchange   _____

Milk	Veg	Fruit	Bread	Meat	Fat
3	4	3	7	8	7

1900-Calorie, Low-Calorie, Low-Carbohydrate Day

Breakfast

    1 ½ bread exchanges   _____
    1 ½ fat exchanges   _____
    2 fruit exchanges   _____
    1 milk exchange   _____

Morning Snack

    1 fruit exchange   _____

Lunch

    3 ½ meat exchanges   _____
    2 ½ bread exchanges   _____
    1 veg exchange   _____
    2 ½ fat exchanges   _____
    1 milk exchange   _____

Afternoon Snack

    ½ bread exchange   _____

Dinner

    5 ½ meat exchanges   _____
    2 bread exchanges   _____
    3 veg exchanges   _____
    3 fat exchanges   _____
    1 milk exchange   _____

Evening Snack

    ½ bread exchange   _____
    1 fruit exchange   _____

Milk	Veg	Fruit	Bread	Meat	Fat
3	4	4	7	9	7

2000-Calorie, Low-Calorie, Low-Carbohydrate Day

Breakfast

    1½ bread exchanges   ——————————

    1½ fat exchanges   ——————————

    2 fruit exchanges   ——————————

    1 milk exchange   ——————————

Morning Snack

    1 fruit exchange   ——————————

Lunch

    3½ meat exchanges   ——————————

    2 bread exchanges   ——————————

    1 veg exchange   ——————————

    3½ fat exchanges   ——————————

    1 milk exchange   ——————————

Afternoon Snack

    1 bread exchange   ——————————

Dinner

    5½ meat exchanges   ——————————

    2½ bread exchanges   ——————————

    3 veg exchanges   ——————————

    3 fat exchanges   ——————————

    1 milk exchange   ——————————

Evening Snack

    1 bread exchange   ——————————

    1 fruit exchange   ——————————

Milk	Veg	Fruit	Bread	Meat	Fat
3	4	4	8	9	8

900-Calorie, High-Calorie, High-Carbohydrate Day

Breakfast

    1 bread exchange   _____

    1 fat exchange   _____

    ½ fruit exchange   _____

    ½ milk exchange   _____

Morning Snack

    1 bread exchange   _____

    ½ fruit exchange   _____

Lunch

    2 bread exchanges   _____

    1 ½ veg exchanges   _____

    1 ½ fat exchanges   _____

Afternoon Snack

    ½ fruit exchange   _____

Dinner

    2 bread exchanges   _____

    1 ½ veg exchanges   _____

    1 ½ fat exchanges   _____

Evening Snack

    ½ fruit exchange   _____

    ½ milk exchange   _____

Milk	Veg	Fruit	Bread	Meat	Fat
1	3	2	6	0	4

1000-Calorie, High-Calorie, High-Carbohydrate Day

Breakfast

    1 bread exchange   _____
    1 fat exchange   _____
    ½ fruit exchange   _____
    ½ milk exchange   _____

Morning Snack

    1 bread exchange   _____
    ½ fruit exchange   _____

Lunch

    2 bread exchanges   _____
    1½ veg exchanges   _____
    2 fat exchanges   _____

Afternoon Snack

    1 fruit exchange   _____

Dinner

    2 bread exchanges   _____
    1½ veg exchanges   _____
    2 fat exchanges   _____

Evening Snack

    1 fruit exchange   _____
    ½ milk exchange   _____

Milk	Veg	Fruit	Bread	Meat	Fat
1	3	2	6	0	5

1100-Calorie, High-Calorie, High-Carbohydrate Day

Breakfast

1 1/2 bread exchanges   _____

1 fat exchange   _____

1/2 fruit exchange   _____

1/2 milk exchange   _____

Morning Snack

1 1/2 bread exchanges   _____

1/2 fruit exchange   _____

Lunch

2 1/2 bread exchanges   _____

1 1/2 veg exchanges   _____

2 fat exchanges   _____

Afternoon Snack

1/2 fruit exchange   _____

Dinner

2 1/2 bread exchanges   _____

1 1/2 veg exchanges   _____

2 fat exchanges   _____

Evening Snack

1/2 fruit exchange   _____

1/2 milk exchange   _____

Milk	Veg	Fruit	Bread	Meat	Fat
1	3	2	8	0	5

1200-Calorie, High-Calorie, High-Carbohydrate Day

Breakfast

    2 bread exchanges   _____

    1 fat exchange   _____

    ½ fruit exchange   _____

    ½ milk exchange   _____

Morning Snack

    2 bread exchanges   _____

    ½ fruit exchange   _____

Lunch

    2½ bread exchanges   _____

    2 veg exchanges   _____

    2 fat exchanges   _____

Afternoon Snack

    ½ fruit exchange   _____

Dinner

    2½ bread exchanges   _____

    2 veg exchanges   _____

    2 fat exchanges   _____

Evening Snack

    ½ fruit exchange   _____

    ½ milk exchange   _____

Milk	Veg	Fruit	Bread	Meat	Fat
1	4	2	9	0	5

1300-Calorie, High-Calorie, High-Carbohydrate Day

Breakfast

    2 bread exchanges   _____

    1 fat exchange   _____

    ½ fruit exchange   _____

    1 milk exchange   _____

Morning Snack

    2 bread exchanges   _____

    ½ fruit exchange   _____

Lunch

    2½ bread exchanges   _____

    1½ veg exchanges   _____

    2½ fat exchanges   _____

Afternoon Snack

    1 fruit exchange   _____

Dinner

    2½ bread exchanges   _____

    1½ veg exchanges   _____

    2½ fat exchanges   _____

Evening Snack

    1 fruit exchange   _____

    1 milk exchange   _____

Milk	Veg	Fruit	Bread	Meat	Fat
2	3	3	9	0	6

1400-Calorie, High-Calorie, High-Carbohydrate Day

Breakfast

    2 bread exchanges   _____

    1 fat exchange   _____

    ½ fruit exchange   _____

    1 milk exchange   _____

Morning Snack

    2 bread exchanges   _____

    ½ fruit exchange   _____

Lunch

    3 bread exchanges   _____

    1½ veg exchanges   _____

    2½ fat exchanges   _____

Afternoon Snack

    1 fruit exchange   _____

Dinner

    3 bread exchanges   _____

    1½ veg exchanges   _____

    2½ fat exchanges   _____

Evening Snack

    1 fruit exchange   _____

    1 milk exchange   _____

Milk	Veg	Fruit	Bread	Meat	Fat
2	3	3	10	0	6

1500-Calorie, High-Calorie, High-Carbohydrate Day

Breakfast

    2 bread exchanges   _____

    1 ½ fat exchanges   _____

    ½ fruit exchange   _____

    1 milk exchange   _____

Morning Snack

    2 bread exchanges   _____

    ½ fruit exchange   _____

Lunch

    3 bread exchanges   _____

    2 veg exchanges   _____

    2 ½ fat exchanges   _____

Afternoon Snack

    1 fruit exchange   _____

Dinner

    3 bread exchanges   _____

    2 veg exchanges   _____

    3 fat exchanges   _____

Evening Snack

    1 fruit exchange   _____

    1 milk exchange   _____

Milk	Veg	Fruit	Bread	Meat	Fat
2	4	3	10	0	7

1600-Calorie, High-Calorie, High-Carbohydrate Day

Breakfast

    2 bread exchanges   _____

    1 ½ fat exchanges   _____

    1 fruit exchange   _____

    1 milk exchange   _____

Morning Snack

    2 bread exchanges   _____

    1 fruit exchange   _____

Lunch

    3 ½ bread exchanges   _____

    2 veg exchanges   _____

    2 ½ fat exchanges   _____

Afternoon Snack

    1 fruit exchange   _____

Dinner

    3 ½ bread exchanges   _____

    2 veg exchanges   _____

    3 fat exchanges   _____

Evening Snack

    1 fruit exchange   _____

    1 milk exchange   _____

Milk	Veg	Fruit	Bread	Meat	Fat
2	4	4	11	0	7

1700-Calorie, High-Calorie, High-Carbohydrate Day

Breakfast

    2½ bread exchanges   _____
    1½ fat exchanges   _____
    1 fruit exchange   _____
    1 milk exchange   _____

Morning Snack

    2½ bread exchanges   _____
    1 fruit exchange   _____

Lunch

    3½ bread exchanges   _____
    2 veg exchanges   _____
    2½ fat exchanges   _____

Afternoon Snack

    1 fruit exchange   _____

Dinner

    3½ bread exchanges   _____
    2 veg exchanges   _____
    3 fat exchanges   _____

Evening Snack

    1 fruit exchange   _____
    1 milk exchange   _____

Milk	Veg	Fruit	Bread	Meat	Fat
2	4	4	12	0	7

1800-Calorie, High-Calorie, High-Carbohydrate Day

Breakfast

    2½ bread exchanges   _____

    1½ fat exchanges   _____

    1 fruit exchange   _____

    1½ milk exchanges   _____

Morning Snack

    2½ bread exchanges   _____

    1 fruit exchange   _____

Lunch

    3½ bread exchanges   _____

    2 veg exchanges   _____

    3½ fat exchanges   _____

Afternoon Snack

    1 fruit exchange   _____

Dinner

    3½ bread exchanges   _____

    2 veg exchanges   _____

    3 fat exchanges   _____

Evening Snack

    1 fruit exchange   _____

    1½ milk exchanges   _____

Milk	Veg	Fruit	Bread	Meat	Fat
3	4	4	12	0	8

1900-Calorie, High-Calorie, High-Carbohydrate Day

Breakfast

    2½ bread exchanges   ————————

    1½ fat exchanges   ————————

    1 fruit exchange   ————————

    1½ milk exchanges   ————————

Morning Snack

    2½ bread exchanges   ————————

    1 fruit exchange   ————————

Lunch

    4 bread exchanges   ————————

    2 veg exchanges   ————————

    3½ fat exchanges   ————————

Afternoon Snack

    1 fruit exchange   ————————

Dinner

    4 bread exchanges   ————————

    2 veg exchanges   ————————

    3 fat exchanges   ————————

Evening Snack

    1 fruit exchange   ————————

    1½ milk exchanges   ————————

Milk	Veg	Fruit	Bread	Meat	Fat
3	4	4	13	0	8

2000-Calorie, High-Calorie, High-Carbohydrate Day

Breakfast

    3 bread exchanges   _____

    2 fat exchanges   _____

    1 fruit exchange   _____

    1 1/2 milk exchanges   _____

Morning Snack

    3 bread exchanges   _____

    1 fruit exchange   _____

Lunch

    4 bread exchanges   _____

    2 veg exchanges   _____

    3 1/2 fat exchanges   _____

Afternoon Snack

    1 fruit exchange   _____

Dinner

    4 bread exchanges   _____

    2 veg exchanges   _____

    3 1/2 fat exchanges   _____

Evening Snack

    1 fruit exchange   _____

    1 1/2 milk exchanges   _____

Milk	Veg	Fruit	Bread	Meat	Fat
3	4	4	14	0	9

2100-Calorie, High-Calorie, High-Carbohydrate Day

Breakfast

    3 bread exchanges   _____

    2 fat exchanges   _____

    2 fruit exchanges   _____

    1 milk exchange   _____

Morning Snack

    1 fruit exchange   _____

Lunch

    4½ bread exchanges   _____

    1½ veg exchanges   _____

    3½ fat exchanges   _____

    1 milk exchange   _____

Afternoon Snack

    1½ bread exchanges   _____

Dinner

    4½ bread exchanges   _____

    3½ veg exchanges   _____

    3½ fat exchanges   _____

    1 milk exchange   _____

Evening Snack

    1½ bread exchanges   _____

    1 fruit exchange   _____

Milk	Veg	Fruit	Bread	Meat	Fat
3	5	4	15	0	9

2200-Calorie, High-Calorie, High-Carbohydrate Day

Breakfast

    3 bread exchanges   _____

    2 fat exchanges   _____

    2 fruit exchanges   _____

    1 milk exchange   _____

Morning Snack

    1 1/2 fruit exchanges   _____

Lunch

    4 1/2 bread exchanges   _____

    1 1/2 veg exchanges   _____

    4 fat exchanges   _____

    1 milk exchange   _____

Afternoon Snack

    1 1/2 bread exchanges   _____

Dinner

    4 1/2 bread exchanges   _____

    3 1/2 veg exchanges   _____

    4 fat exchanges   _____

    1 milk exchange   _____

Evening Snack

    1 1/2 bread exchanges   _____

    1 1/2 fruit exchanges   _____

Milk	Veg	Fruit	Bread	Meat	Fat
3	5	5	15	0	10

2300-Calorie, High-Calorie, High-Carbohydrate Day

Breakfast

    3 bread exchanges   _____

    2 fat exchanges   _____

    2 fruit exchanges   _____

    1 milk exchange   _____

Morning Snack

    1 1/2 fruit exchanges   _____

Lunch

    4 1/2 bread exchanges   _____

    1 1/2 veg exchanges   _____

    4 fat exchanges   _____

    1 milk exchange   _____

Afternoon Snack

    1 1/2 bread exchanges   _____

Dinner

    4 1/2 bread exchanges   _____

    3 1/2 veg exchanges   _____

    4 fat exchanges   _____

    2 milk exchanges   _____

Evening Snack

    1 1/2 bread exchanges   _____

    1 1/2 fruit exchanges   _____

Milk	Veg	Fruit	Bread	Meat	Fat
4	5	5	15	0	10

2400-Calorie, High-Calorie, High-Carbohydrate Day

Breakfast

    3 bread exchanges   _____

    2 fat exchanges   _____

    2 fruit exchanges   _____

    1 milk exchange   _____

Morning Snack

    1½ fruit exchanges   _____

Lunch

    5 bread exchanges   _____

    1½ veg exchanges   _____

    4 fat exchanges   _____

    1 milk exchange   _____

Afternoon Snack

    1½ bread exchanges   _____

Dinner

    5 bread exchanges   _____

    3½ veg exchanges   _____

    4 fat exchanges   _____

    2 milk exchanges   _____

Evening Snack

    1½ bread exchanges   _____

    1½ fruit exchanges   _____

Milk	Veg	Fruit	Bread	Meat	Fat
4	5	5	16	0	10

2500-Calorie, High-Calorie, High-Carbohydrate Day

Breakfast

    3 bread exchanges   _____

    2 fat exchanges   _____

    2 fruit exchanges   _____

    1 milk exchange   _____

Morning Snack

    1½ fruit exchanges   _____

Lunch

    5 bread exchanges   _____

    1½ veg exchanges   _____

    4½ fat exchanges   _____

    1 milk exchange   _____

Afternoon Snack

    1½ bread exchanges   _____

Dinner

    5 bread exchanges   _____

    3½ veg exchanges   _____

    4½ fat exchanges   _____

    2 milk exchanges   _____

Evening Snack

    1½ bread exchanges   _____

    1½ fruit exchanges   _____

Milk	Veg	Fruit	Bread	Meat	Fat
4	5	5	16	0	11

APPENDIX B.
THE PRINCETON PLAN FOR
STRICT VEGETARIANS

THE basic Princeton Plan for weight loss alternates low-carbohydrate days on which some meat is eaten with high-carbohydrate, essentially vegetarian days. Meat, poultry, and fish are included in the basic plan because they contain a number of essential nutrients that cannot easily be obtained through nonmeat sources. Nevertheless, with care, the Princeton Plan can be adapted to a strict vegetarian regimen.

The following chart shows vegetable sources of omega-3 fatty acids. The charts on pages 281–284 provide sample menu plans for vegetarian reducing diets. (When choosing "meat" exchanges, select nonanimal proteins such as tofu and nuts.)

VEGETABLE SOURCES OF
OMEGA-3 FATTY ACIDS

(Grams of Omega-3 Fatty Acids
Per 3.5-Ounce Portion)

Butternuts	11.1
Walnuts	6.8
Black walnuts	3.3
Soy sprouts	2.1
Soybeans (dried)	1.6
Hickory nuts	1.0
Wheat germ	.7
Navy or pinto beans	.6
Purslane	.3
Lima beans	.2
Dried peas	.2

*Note that omega-3 fatty acids from plant
sources may not be as easily used in the
body as omega-3s from animal sources.

Strict Vegetarian
1000-Calorie, Low-Calorie, Low-Carbohydrate Day

Breakfast

    ½ bread exchange   _____

    ½ fat exchange   _____

    1 fruit exchange   _____

Morning Snack

    1 fruit exchange   _____

Lunch

    2½ meat exchanges   _____

    1 bread exchange   _____

    1 veg exchange   _____

    1 fat exchange   _____

    1 fruit exchange   _____

Afternoon Snack

    ½ bread exchange   _____

Dinner

    4 meat exchanges   _____

    1 bread exchange   _____

    3 veg exchanges   _____

    1 fat exchange

Milk	Veg	Fruit	Bread	Meat	Fat
0	4	3	3	6½	2½

Strict Vegetarian
1400-Calorie, High-Calorie, High-Carbohydrate Day

Breakfast

    3 bread exchanges   _____
    1 fat exchange   _____
    1 fruit exchange   _____

Morning Snack

    1 fruit exchange   _____

Lunch

    1 meat exchange   _____
    3 ½ bread exchanges   _____
    1 veg exchange   _____
    2 fat exchanges   _____
    1 fruit exchange   _____

Afternoon Snack

    1 bread exchange   _____

Dinner

    1 meat exchange   _____
    3 ½ bread exchanges   _____
    2 veg exchanges   _____
    2 fat exchanges

Milk	Veg	Fruit	Bread	Meat	Fat
0	3	3	11	2	5

Strict Vegetarian
1200-Calorie, Low-Calorie, Low-Carbohydrate Day

Breakfast

    1 ½ bread exchanges   _____
    ½ fat exchange   _____
    2 fruit exchanges   _____

Morning Snack

    1 fruit exchange   _____

Lunch

    3 meat exchanges   _____
    1 bread exchange   _____
    1 ½ veg exchanges   _____
    1 ½ fat exchanges   _____
    1 fruit exchange   _____

Afternoon Snack

    ½ bread exchange   _____

Dinner

    5 meat exchanges   _____
    1 bread exchange   _____
    3 ½ veg exchanges   _____
    1 fat exchange

Milk	Veg	Fruit	Bread	Meat	Fat
0	5	4	4	8	3

Strict Vegetarian
1700-Calorie, High-Calorie, High-Carbohydrate Day

Breakfast

    3 bread exchanges   _____

    1 fat exchange   _____

    2 fruit exchanges   _____

Morning Snack

    1 fruit exchange   _____

Lunch

    1 meat exchange   _____

    4 bread exchanges   _____

    1½ veg exchanges   _____

    2½ fat exchanges   _____

    1 fruit exchange   _____

Afternoon Snack

    1½ bread exchanges   _____

Dinner

    1½ meat exchanges   _____

    4 bread exchanges   _____

    3½ veg exchanges   _____

    2½ fat exchanges

Milk	Veg	Fruit	Bread	Meat	Fat
0	5	4	12½	2½	6

APPENDIX C.
THE PRINCETON PLAN FOR MEAT LOVERS

THE following plans provide sample menus for a Princeton Plan reducing diet in which limited amounts of meat are allowed on the high-carbohydrate, high-calorie day as well as on the low-carbohydrate, low-calorie day.

Note that even if no milk is used on the high-carbohydrate day, which allows more exchanges of protein to be used, there is still very little meat (one or two exchanges) that can be eaten on that day.

Meat on "Vegetarian" Day
1400-Calorie, High-Calorie, High-Carbohydrate Day

Breakfast

    3 bread exchanges   ————————————
    1 fat exchange   ————————————
    1 fruit exchange   ————————————

Morning Snack

    1 fruit exchange   ————————————

Lunch

    ½ meat exchange   ————————————
    3 bread exchanges   ————————————
    1 veg exchange   ————————————
    2½ fat exchanges   ————————————
    1 fruit exchange   ————————————

Afternoon Snack

    1 bread exchange   ————————————

Dinner

    1 meat exchange   ————————————
    3 bread exchanges   ————————————
    3 veg exchanges   ————————————
    2 fat exchanges

Milk	Veg	Fruit	Bread	Meat	Fat
0	4	3	10	1½	5½

Meat on "Vegetarian" Day
1700-Calorie, High-Calorie, High-Carbohydrate Day

Breakfast

    4 bread exchanges   _____

    1 ½ fat exchanges   _____

    1 fruit exchange   _____

Morning Snack

    1 fruit exchange   _____

Lunch

    1 meat exchange   _____

    4 bread exchanges   _____

    1 veg exchange   _____

    2 ½ fat exchanges   _____

    1 fruit exchange   _____

Afternoon Snack

    1 bread exchanges   _____

Dinner

    1 meat exchange   _____

    4 bread exchanges   _____

    3 veg exchanges   _____

    2 ½ fat exchanges

Milk	Veg	Fruit	Bread	Meat	Fat
0	4	3	13	2	6 ½

APPENDIX D.
ABSTRACT: PROSTAGLANDINS, BROWN FAT, AND WEIGHT LOSS*

E. P. HELENIAK, M.D., AND B. ASTON, M.S.

IN obesity, a situation is created in which energy intake exceeds energy expenditure. The three components of energy expenditure are resting metabolism, physical activity, and thermogenesis. Increasing attention is being paid to the role of impaired energy expenditure in obesity. Evidence indicates that impairment in activity of the sympathetic nervous system, which stimulates thermogenic processes, contributes to the etiology of obesity. In addition, insulin resistance, a well-recognized metabolic consequence of obesity, appears to interfere with feeding-related, insulin-mediated increases in thermogenesis in brown adipose tissue. This thermogenic defect results in reduced energy buffering by brown adipose tissue leading to deficient energy expenditure and an increased efficiency in weight gain. A unique weight loss program, The Princeton Metabolic Diet Program, is presented. The Program stimulates metabolism by stimulating the sympathetic nervous system and correcting insulin resistance, thereby

Medical Hypotheses (1989) 28, 13–33, © Longman Group UK Ltd 1989.

The complete paper may be ordered from The Princeton Brain Bio Center, 862 Route 518, Skillman, NJ 08558. Reader must send a self-addressed, stamped, 9 1/2- by 4-inch business envelope. Postage required is for two ounces.

enhancing thermogenesis in brown adipose tissue. Methods include: 1) alternating diet composition and caloric intake and, 2) the use of nutritional metabolic stimulants. This type of non-toxic therapy, directed at correcting biochemical defects, will enhance metabolic mechanisms and induce weight loss.

SELECTED BIBLIOGRAPHY

THE following are popular books providing further information on aerobic and strength-building exercises.

Cooper, Kenneth. *The New Aerobics.* New York: Bantam, 1984. Paper, $4.50.

Darden, Elliot. *The Nautilus Book,* rev. ed. New York: Contemporary Books, 1985. Paper, $9.95.

Reynolds, Bill. *The Complete Weight Training Book.* Mountain View, California: Anderson World, 1979. Paper, $4.95.

The following books offer more information on various aspects of nutrition and supplementation.

Braverman, Eric R., M.D., with Carl C. Pfeiffer, M.D., Ph.D. *The Healing Nutrients Within: Facts, Findings, and New Research on Amino Acids.* New Canaan, CT: Keats, 1987. Cloth, $23.95.

Erasmus, Udo. *Fats and Oils: The Complete Guide to Fats and Oils in Health and Nutrition.* Burnaby, B.C., Canada: Alive Books, 1986. Paper, U.S. $16.50.

Horrobin, David F., ed. *Clinical Uses of Essential Fatty Acids.* Montreal: Eden Press, 1982. Cloth, $35.

Pfeiffer, Carl C., M.D., Ph.D. *Mental and Elemental Nutrients: A Physician's Guide to Nutrition and Health Care.* New Canaan, CT: Keats, 1976. Cloth, $14.95.

The following periodicals provide a layperson's guide to the latest in medical, nutritional, and exercise news.

Let's Live. 444 N. Larchmont Blvd., Box 74908, Los Angeles, CA 74908. Monthly; one-year subscription $9.95. Focuses mainly on nutrition; each issue contains a number of healthful recipes.

Nutrition Action Healthletter. Published by the Center for Science in the Public Interest, 1501 16th St., N.W., Washington, D.C., 20036-1499. A one-year membership in CSPI, a nonprofit group devoted to improved health and nutrition, includes ten issues of the excellent *Healthletter.*

Prevention. Rodale Press, 33 East Minor Street, Erasmus, PA 18049. A one-year subscription is $15.97. This monthly magazine is devoted to healthy living, nutrition, and exercise.

INDEX